C
ADDICT'S
CARBOHYDRATE
COUNTER

D0372536

THE CARBOHYDRATE ADDICT'S CARBOHYDRATE COUNTER

DR. RACHAEL F. HELLER

ASSISTANT PROFESSOR EMERITUS, MT. SINAI SCHOOL OF MEDICINE•
ASSISTANT PROFESSOR EMERITUS, GRADUATE CENTER OF THE
CITY UNIVERSITY OF NEW YORK

DR. RICHARD F. HELLER

PROFESSOR EMERITUS, MT. SINAI SCHOOL OF MEDICINE•
PROFESSOR EMERITUS, GRADUATE CENTER OF THE
CITY UNIVERSITY OF NEW YORK•
PROFESSOR EMERITUS, CITY UNIVERSITY OF NEW YORK

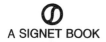

A SIGNET BOOK

A Note to the Reader
The ideas and data contained in this book are not intended as a substitute for
medical treatment by a physician. The reader should regularly consult a physician
in matters relating to health and prior to any change in diet.

SIGNET
Published by New American Library, a division of
Penguin Putnam Inc., 375 Hudson Street,
New York, New York 10014, U.S.A.
Penguin Books Ltd, 27 Wrights Lane, London W8 5TZ, England
Penguin Books Australia Ltd, Ringwood, Victoria, Australia
Penguin Books Canada Ltd, 10 Alcorn Avenue, Toronto, Ontario, Canada M4V 3B2
Penguin Books (N.Z.) Ltd, 182–190 Wairau Road, Auckland 10, New Zealand

Penguin Books Ltd, Registered Offices
Harmondsworth, Middlesex, England

First published by Signet, an imprint of New American Library,
a division of Penguin Putnam Inc.

First Printing, January 2000
10   9

REGISTERED TRADEMARK—MARCA REGISTRADA

Printed in the United States of America

CONTENTS

In this counter you will find more than **4000 food comparisons*** presented in two exciting, easy and reader-friendly formats. The major categories and the page numbers on which you will find them are as follows:

*Nutritional values in this counter were taken from material supplied by or direct communication with the U.S. Department of Agriculture, scientific studies, computer data banks, and representatives of the food industry. When counts, as provided by a variety of sources, differ one from the other, an average or typical count is calculated and used. All data are rounded to the nearest whole number. Neither the authors nor publisher assume any responsibility for any errors contained herein and all readers must work in accordance with and in conjunction with their own personal physician. For information on abbreviations, see the introductory pages that follow.

INTRODUCTION

Are You a Carbohydrate Addict?

Do you find that once you start to eat breads and other starches, snack foods or sweets, you have a very difficult time stopping? Do you eat too much of these carbohydrate-rich foods—even though you said you would "control" yourself? If so, it is likely that you are a carbohydrate addict. Your body may respond differently to that bread or pasta or potato, to those snack foods or sweets, than do other people.

As in many things, science is starting to realize that we are individuals and we differ in the way we respond to foods. C. Everett Koop, M.D., the former Surgeon General of the United States, calls us "carbohydrate sensitive." Researchers have shown that as many as 75 percent of the overweight (and many normal-weight individuals as well) appear to have a physical imbalance that leads to an addiction to carbohydrates.

This physical imbalance, an imbalance in the hormone insulin, makes us crave carbohydrate-rich foods intensely and repeatedly and we are more likely to put on weight and to keep it on. Our genes have made carbohydrate-rich foods taste better, made us extraordinarily good at storing away carbohydrates in the form of fat, and no matter how great our willpower, our bodies seem to fight us at every level.

It is important to understand that carbohydrate addiction is not a matter of willpower but rather a matter of biology. If you are a carbohydrate addict, your cravings and your weight gain are symptoms of an underlying physical imbalance; we know what causes it and, best of all, we now know how to correct it.

If you are a carbohydrate addict, you may find that:

- After you've had a full breakfast, you get hungrier before it's time for lunch

- You have difficulty stopping once you've started to eat bread, pasta or other starches, snack foods or sweets
- You get tired and/or hungry in the mid-afternoon and a snack makes you feel better
- You may put weight on easily or, after dieting, tend to gain it back quickly
- You sometimes lose control of your eating
- You continue to eat or snack even when you are not hungry

If you are addicted to carbohydrates, we understand why you have struggled to stay on diets and why diets often fail to help you keep the weight off. Carbohydrate-rich foods may hold the key to your addiction and to your success.

On our Programs, you can enjoy these foods every day, in satisfying and pleasurable quantities, while working within our guidelines. For our Programs' essential guidelines, see *The Carbohydrate Addict's LifeSpan Program* (Plume), *The Carbohydrate Addict's Healthy for Life Plan* (Plume), *The Carbohydrate Addict's Diet* (Signet) or *The Carbohydrate Addict's Healthy Heart Program* (Ballantine). Our companion workbook, *The Carbohydrate Addict's Program for Success* (Plume), offers help with the emotional and spiritual aspects of carbohydrate addiction, and our other *Carbohydrate Addict's Counters* (Signet) of graphically formatted information charts can provide vital facts for success.

From the Authors: A Special Message

As kids and teens we were both overweight. Not surprisingly, we became overweight adults. The caloric content of foods was as familiar to us as any school subject. And, through the years, each of us had struggled to understand the calorie counters that were available to help us track and get control of our energy intake.

One thing we agree on: the calorie counters of our childhood were barely usable. They were little more than uninteresting little books, filled with never-ending columns and rows of tiny numbers that were a chore to use and often ended up in some bureau drawer or under the couch pillows.

With the advent of gram counters, we attempted to keep track of our carbohydrate and fat levels, only to be confronted with the same boring and unrewarding columns and rows of numbers. To make matters worse, we found ourselves facing the almost impossible task of making an informed choice when the data in these counters were reporting on widely varying amounts. The carbohydrate content of a cup of one soup was listed next to the carbohydrate content of an entire can of another. In some cases, one soup had been diluted; in other cases, the count was based on soup that was still condensed. While we understood that this noncomparable listing was easier and faster for the author, we also knew that it made things far more difficult—if not impossible—for us as readers.

More often than not, we found ourselves using these gram counters less and less frequently until they, too, ended up discarded or lost. Inevitably, we blamed ourselves for not being disciplined enough. In the end, we realized that the very counter we were using was leaving us confused, frustrated, and unmotivated.

Like us, many people have come to expect that gram counting is a tedious but necessary activity for health-risk reduction and weight loss. Not true! We think that you will soon see that gram counting can be fun, simple, and very rewarding. You'll find yourself saying to friends, "Did you know that . . ." and you will enjoy having a handle on your choices, perhaps for the first time in your life.

In the books that make up our Carbohydrate Addict's Counters series, information on the calorie, carbohydrate, and fat content of foods, respectively, are simple to see and easy to compare.

You will be able to walk into a fast food restaurant or down your favorite supermarket aisle and feel like you are in control—because you will be. You will be able to make carbohydrate-related choices in an instant and feel free of nagging doubts and guilt.

And you will grow more confident with each success you achieve.

We have lost more than a combined two hundred pounds between us and we have maintained our ideal weight and health for over fifteen years. We are happier, healthier, and more energetic than we ever were in our twenties or thirties.

Our wish is that you, too, discover the joy that comes as the challenges of the past are replaced by successes of the present (and future). All the struggles that have gone before fade in the face of today's victories.

With our warmest wishes,
Drs. Richard and Rachael Heller

Two Paths to Success

You are about to discover two unique, fun, and easy formats for gram counting; two types of charts will help put you in charge of making your carbohydrate-related food choices.

The first new format you will discover has been used in our Alphabetical Charts. They can be found in the front half of this book. Alphabetical charts list foods from A to Z and allow you to locate a specific food item by its name, within its food group.

Alphabetical Charts will make it easy for you to see, at a glance, how carbohydrate-dense your food choice is, as compared to other foods within that same group. Alphabetical Charts will help you to decide if the carbohydrate level of food makes it a good selection for you. In addition to the bars that illustrate the amount of carbohydrates in each food, the number at the end of each bar will provide you with specific levels of carbohydrate content.

In the second half of this book you will find Hi-Low Comparison Charts, a second type of chart to help you compare foods within a given group and visualize foods with regard to their carbohydrate count—from high to low and all those in between.

Hi-Low Comparison Charts can be wonderful tools when

you want some suggestions on what to eat while keeping your carbohydrate goals in mind.

What Is a Carbohydrate?

Carbohydrates are one of the three macronutrients (large nutrients) needed by the body in order to repair, fuel, and maintain itself. Most carbohydrates are from plant sources and include all types of sugars, starches, and dietary fiber.

Simple carbohydrates are sugars. These are found in many foods, including apples to yogurt, soups and fruits and juices, and sugary foods including candy and soda. Sugars usually have an "ose" ending, as in glucose, fructose, and sucrose.

Complex carbohydrates are actually simple sugars strung together like pearls on a string, forming a necklace. Complex carbohydrates are preferred as a source of nutrition because they are less likely to cause blood sugar swings and because they are usually higher in fiber and richer in vitamins and minerals as well. Complex carbohydrates are found in grains, rice, pasta, and starchy vegetables such as corn and potatoes. Although legumes are high in protein they are also high in carbohydrates.

Scientists are continuing to discover the importance of fiber, another type of carbohydrate that is very important to a healthful diet. Although many people refer to fiber as if it were a single entity, many foods supply different kinds of fiber. Fiber is divided into two main groups, soluble and insoluble. Insoluble fiber does not dissolve in water and cannot be broken down by stomach acid, so it moves quickly through the gastrointestinal tract and promotes the swift elimination of fecal matter. Insoluble fiber has been shown to relieve constipation and prevent hemorrhoids and appears to be very important in reducing risk for colon cancer. As your physician recommends, insoluble fiber may be an important adjunct to your eating program. Insoluble-fiber-rich foods include fruits, vegetables, and wholewheat products, including wheat bran.

Soluble fiber, on the other hand, dissolves in water (even though it remains intact while inside the body). In the intestines, soluble fiber forms a jelly-like mass that binds with cholesterol and appears to promote its excretion from the body. Due to its binding effect, soluble fiber has a powerful cholesterol-lowering effect, reducing both total cholesterol and low-density blood fats, important actions that may help reduce your risk for heart disease.

Soluble fiber has been shown to help balance insulin levels and improve sugar metabolism as well.

Soluble fiber can be found in beans, oats, barley, soybeans, fruits, and vegetables. It is always best to get your fiber from your food. While soluble fiber can also be found in psyllium seed, pectin, and guar gum, the use of concentrated fiber supplementation from these high-fiber sources is not recommended unless your physician thinks it necessary.

How Much Carbohydrate Do I Need?

According to The American Heart Association's Eating Plan for Healthy Americans, carbohydrates should make up 55–60 percent or more of calories, with an emphasis on increasing sources of complex carbohydrates. Each gram of carbohydrate contains approximately 4 calories. For your particular needs, consult with your physician.

Am I Overweight?

While there is no definitive way to determine whether you are at your ideal weight, here are three ways to help you in your evaluation.

Weight Check #1: The Chart

The chart that follows is a standardized chart used by the United States Department of Agriculture.

Weight Check #2: The Pinch

Weight range charts can help you to determine whether you have a weight problem but they don't necessarily tell you the whole story. What may look quite acceptable on the scale may look different to the well-trained eye. Likewise, an "over-

RANGE OF "DESIRABLE" WEIGHTS*

Height without shoes	Weight without clothes	
	Men (pounds)	Women (pounds)
4'10"		92–121
4'11"		95–124
5'0"		98–127
5'1"	105–134	101–130
5'2"	108–137	104–134
5'3"	111–141	107–138
5'4"	114–145	110–142
5'5"	117–149	114–146
5'6"	121–154	118–150
5'7"	125–159	122–154
5'8"	129–163	126–159
5'9"	133–167	130–164
5'10"	137–172	134–169
5'11"	141–177	
6'0"	145–182	
6'1"	149–187	
6'2"	153–192	
6'3"	157–197	

*United States Department of Agriculture Human Nutrition Information Service Agriculture, Information Bulletin 364.

weight" person may be perfectly fit and in good condition depending on his or her muscle mass.

If you want to try a simple and quick test, pinch a fold of skin at the back of your upper arm. If you can pinch more than an inch, you are probably carrying more weight (in the form of fat) than is desirable.

Weight Check #3: Body Mass Index (BMI)

Body Mass Index Scores appear to provide a better picture of an individual's weight level. Using a mathematical formula, the BMI takes into account both a person's weight and height. BMI equals a person's weight in kilograms divided by height in meters squared (BMI=kg/m²). We'll keep it simple! The table that follows will make it easy for you to get your BMI score.

To use the BMI table that follows, find your height in the left-hand column. Move across the row to your weight. The number at the bottom of the column is your Body Mass Index (BMI).

BODY MASS INDEX (BMI) CHART

Height (in.)

58	91	96	100	105	110	115	119	124	129	134	138	143	167	191
59	94	99	104	109	114	119	124	128	133	138	143	148	173	198
60	97	102	107	112	118	123	128	133	138	143	148	153	179	204
61	100	106	111	116	122	127	132	137	143	148	153	158	185	211
62	104	109	115	120	126	131	136	142	147	153	158	164	191	218
63	107	113	118	124	130	135	141	146	152	158	163	169	197	225
64	110	116	122	128	134	140	145	151	157	163	169	174	204	232
65	114	120	126	132	138	144	150	156	162	168	174	180	210	240
66	118	124	130	136	142	148	155	161	167	173	179	186	216	247
67	121	127	134	140	146	153	159	166	172	178	185	191	223	255
68	125	131	138	144	151	158	164	171	177	184	190	197	230	262
69	128	135	142	149	155	162	169	176	182	189	196	203	236	270
70	132	139	146	153	160	167	174	181	188	195	202	207	243	278
71	136	143	150	157	165	172	179	186	193	200	208	215	250	286
72	140	147	154	162	169	177	184	191	199	206	213	221	258	294
73	144	151	159	166	174	182	189	197	204	212	219	227	265	302
74	148	155	163	171	179	186	194	202	210	218	225	233	272	311
75	152	160	168	176	184	192	200	208	216	224	232	240	279	319
76	156	164	172	180	189	197	205	213	221	230	238	246	287	328
BMI (kg/m²)	19	20	21	22	23	24	25	26	27	28	29	30	35	40

Using your BMI score, the chart below can help you to better determine your weight level.

BMI (Body Mass Index)	Weight Assessment
18.5 or less	Underweight
18.5–24.9	Normal
25.0–29.9	Overweight
30.0–39.9	Obese
40 or greater	Extremely Obese

WHAT REALLY COUNTS

It is our sincerest hope that with the help of this little book, you will find a whole new world of excitement and motivation, good health and success. May the answers you find here bring joy to your life and peace to your heart.

The information that you find in this book may offer you guidance in choosing foods to best meet your health and weight-loss goals. Of all the important tools that are available to you, however, the most important by far is the commitment you bring to making your dreams come true.

So choose the best foods for you, plan and prepare healthful meals and, as appropriate, keep count of the carbohydrates you consume. But in the counting, make certain to count on yourself—your strength, your love of life, and your desire to make your body and your life happy and healthy. You are your most important resource.

ABBREVIATIONS YOU'LL FIND IN
THE CARBOHYDRATE ADDICT'S COUNTERS

When You See This Abbreviation. . . .	It Means This
/	or
w/	with
bl cheese	blue cheese
broc	broccoli
ch	cheese
dress	dressing
env	envelope
fl	fluid or flavor
flav	flavor(s)
Fr dress	French dressing
frzn	frozen
G'ma's Big	Grandma's Big
marg	margarine
parm	parmesan
Pepperidge	Pepperidge Farm
pkg	package
pkt	packet
q'tr pnd'r	quarter pounder
reg	regular
saus	sausage
Stella D	Stella D'Oro
sweet'd	sweetened
Thous Island	Thousand Island
tom	tomato
veg	vegetable
wh	white

THE
CARBOHYDRATE
ADDICT'S
CARBOHYDRATE
COUNTER

ALPHABETICAL CHARTS

BEVERAGES*, Part 1

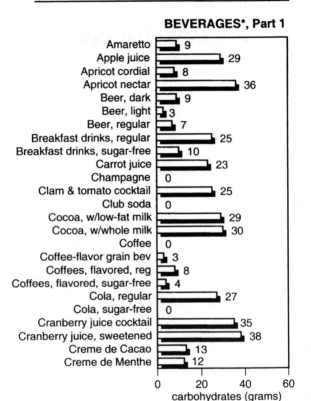

Beverage	carbohydrates (grams)
Amaretto	9
Apple juice	29
Apricot cordial	8
Apricot nectar	36
Beer, dark	9
Beer, light	3
Beer, regular	7
Breakfast drinks, regular	25
Breakfast drinks, sugar-free	10
Carrot juice	23
Champagne	0
Clam & tomato cocktail	25
Club soda	0
Cocoa, w/low-fat milk	29
Cocoa, w/whole milk	30
Coffee	0
Coffee-flavor grain bev	3
Coffees, flavored, reg	8
Coffees, flavored, sugar-free	4
Cola, regular	27
Cola, sugar-free	0
Cranberry juice cocktail	35
Cranberry juice, sweetened	38
Creme de Cacao	13
Creme de Menthe	12

carbohydrates (grams)

* Counts for non-alcoholic drinks and beer are based on
8-fluid-ounce servings, for wine on 3 1/2-fluid-ounce
servings and, for hard liquor, on 1 1/2-fluid-ounce servings.

Alphabetical Chart
(for Hi-Low Comparison Charts, see pages 83 - 164)

BEVERAGES*, Part 2

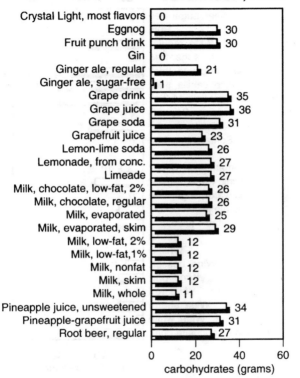

Beverage	carbohydrates (grams)
Crystal Light, most flavors	0
Eggnog	30
Fruit punch drink	30
Gin	0
Ginger ale, regular	21
Ginger ale, sugar-free	1
Grape drink	35
Grape juice	36
Grape soda	31
Grapefruit juice	23
Lemon-lime soda	26
Lemonade, from conc.	27
Limeade	27
Milk, chocolate, low-fat, 2%	26
Milk, chocolate, regular	26
Milk, evaporated	25
Milk, evaporated, skim	29
Milk, low-fat, 2%	12
Milk, low-fat, 1%	12
Milk, nonfat	12
Milk, skim	12
Milk, whole	11
Pineapple juice, unsweetened	34
Pineapple-grapefruit juice	31
Root beer, regular	27

carbohydrates (grams)

* Counts for non-alcoholic drinks and beer are based on
   8-fluid-ounce servings, for wine on 3 1/2-fluid-ounce
   servings and, for hard liquor, on 1 1/2-fluid-ounce servings.

3

BEVERAGES*, Part 3

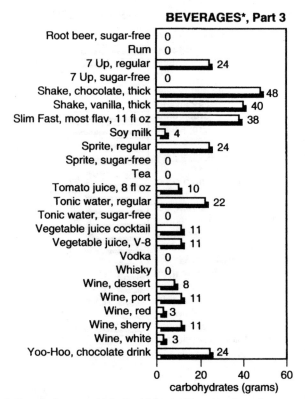

Beverage	carbohydrates (grams)
Root beer, sugar-free	0
Rum	0
7 Up, regular	24
7 Up, sugar-free	0
Shake, chocolate, thick	48
Shake, vanilla, thick	40
Slim Fast, most flav, 11 fl oz	38
Soy milk	4
Sprite, regular	24
Sprite, sugar-free	0
Tea	0
Tomato juice, 8 fl oz	10
Tonic water, regular	22
Tonic water, sugar-free	0
Vegetable juice cocktail	11
Vegetable juice, V-8	11
Vodka	0
Whisky	0
Wine, dessert	8
Wine, port	11
Wine, red	3
Wine, sherry	11
Wine, white	3
Yoo-Hoo, chocolate drink	24

carbohydrates (grams)

* Counts for non-alcoholic drinks and beer are based on
8-fluid-ounce servings, for wine on 3 1/2-fluid-ounce
servings and, for hard liquor, on 1 1/2-fluid-ounce servings.

Bread, Crackers, and Flours:
BAGELS*

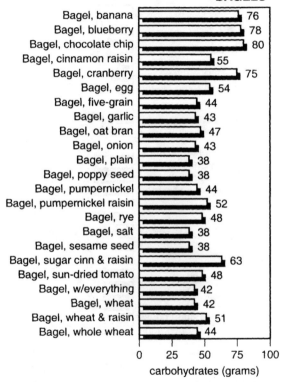

Bagel type	carbohydrates (grams)
Bagel, banana	76
Bagel, blueberry	78
Bagel, chocolate chip	80
Bagel, cinnamon raisin	55
Bagel, cranberry	75
Bagel, egg	54
Bagel, five-grain	44
Bagel, garlic	43
Bagel, oat bran	47
Bagel, onion	43
Bagel, plain	38
Bagel, poppy seed	38
Bagel, pumpernickel	44
Bagel, pumpernickel raisin	52
Bagel, rye	48
Bagel, salt	38
Bagel, sesame seed	38
Bagel, sugar cinn & raisin	63
Bagel, sun-dried tomato	48
Bagel, w/everything	42
Bagel, wheat	42
Bagel, wheat & raisin	51
Bagel, whole wheat	44

carbohydrates (grams)

* Counts are based on one bagel, approximate weight:
3 ounces.

5

Bread, Crackers, and Flours:
BISCUITS, ROLLS & MUFFINS*

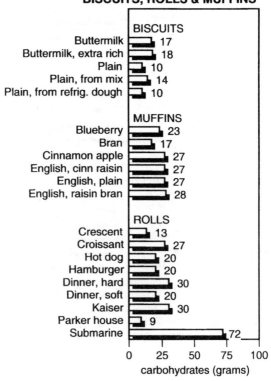

BISCUITS

Buttermilk	17
Buttermilk, extra rich	18
Plain	10
Plain, from mix	14
Plain, from refrig. dough	10

MUFFINS

Blueberry	23
Bran	17
Cinnamon apple	27
English, cinn raisin	27
English, plain	27
English, raisin bran	28

ROLLS

Crescent	13
Croissant	27
Hot dog	20
Hamburger	20
Dinner, hard	30
Dinner, soft	20
Kaiser	30
Parker house	9
Submarine	72

0   25   50   75   100
carbohydrates (grams)

* Counts are based on single, average-size items. Average
sweet muffin is assumed to be 2 3/4 inches by 2 inches.
Average sweet and English muffin weight is 57 grams.

Bread, Crackers, and Flours: BREAD*

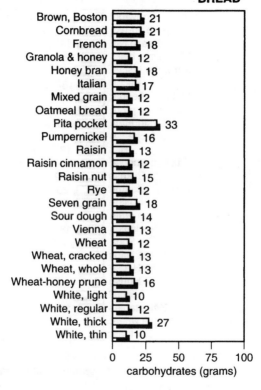

	carbohydrates (grams)
Brown, Boston	21
Cornbread	21
French	18
Granola & honey	12
Honey bran	18
Italian	17
Mixed grain	12
Oatmeal bread	12
Pita pocket	33
Pumpernickel	16
Raisin	13
Raisin cinnamon	12
Raisin nut	15
Rye	12
Seven grain	18
Sour dough	14
Vienna	13
Wheat	12
Wheat, cracked	13
Wheat, whole	13
Wheat-honey prune	16
White, light	10
White, regular	12
White, thick	27
White, thin	10

* Counts are based on one single, average-size slice.

Bread, Crackers, and Flours: CRACKERS*

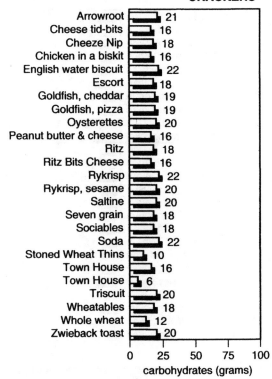

Cracker	carbohydrates (grams)
Arrowroot	21
Cheese tid-bits	16
Cheeze Nip	18
Chicken in a biskit	16
English water biscuit	22
Escort	18
Goldfish, cheddar	19
Goldfish, pizza	19
Oysterettes	20
Peanut butter & cheese	16
Ritz	18
Ritz Bits Cheese	16
Rykrisp	22
Rykrisp, sesame	20
Saltine	20
Seven grain	18
Sociables	18
Soda	22
Stoned Wheat Thins	10
Town House	16
Town House	6
Triscuit	20
Wheatables	18
Whole wheat	12
Zwieback toast	20

carbohydrates (grams)

* For ease of comparison, counts are based on one-ounce
servings. Adjust counts to reflect quantities consumed.

8

Bread, Crackers, and Flours:
DRY & CRISPY

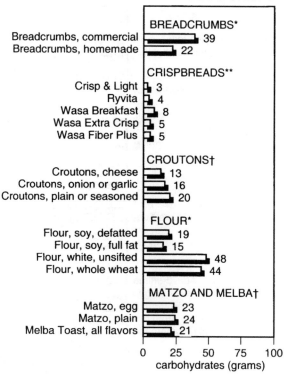

BREADCRUMBS*

Breadcrumbs, commercial — 39
Breadcrumbs, homemade — 22

CRISPBREADS**

Crisp & Light — 3
Ryvita — 4
Wasa Breakfast — 8
Wasa Extra Crisp — 5
Wasa Fiber Plus — 5

CROUTONS†

Croutons, cheese — 13
Croutons, onion or garlic — 16
Croutons, plain or seasoned — 20

FLOUR*

Flour, soy, defatted — 19
Flour, soy, full fat — 15
Flour, white, unsifted — 48
Flour, whole wheat — 44

MATZO AND MELBA†

Matzo, egg — 23
Matzo, plain — 24
Melba Toast, all flavors — 21

0   25   50   75   100
carbohydrates (grams)

* Counts are based on 1/2- cup servings.

** Counts are based on single item.

† Counts are based on single-ounce servings.

Bread, Crackers, and Flours:
PANCAKES, STUFFING & MORE*

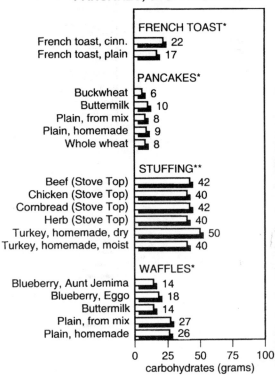

FRENCH TOAST*

French toast, cinn.	22
French toast, plain	17

PANCAKES*

Buckwheat	6
Buttermilk	10
Plain, from mix	8
Plain, homemade	9
Whole wheat	8

STUFFING**

Beef (Stove Top)	42
Chicken (Stove Top)	40
Cornbread (Stove Top)	42
Herb (Stove Top)	40
Turkey, homemade, dry	50
Turkey, homemade, moist	40

WAFFLES*

Blueberry, Aunt Jemima	14
Blueberry, Eggo	18
Buttermilk	14
Plain, from mix	27
Plain, homemade	26

0   25   50   75   100
carbohydrates (grams)

* Counts are based on a single slice, one pancake, or
   one waffle.

** Counts are based on 1/2-cup servings, prepared.

Alphabetical Chart
(for Hi-Low Comparison Charts, see pages 83 - 164)

CEREALS*, Part 1

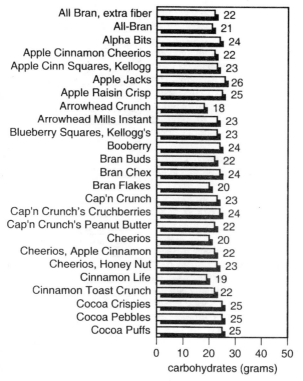

Cereal	carbohydrates (grams)
All Bran, extra fiber	22
All-Bran	21
Alpha Bits	24
Apple Cinnamon Cheerios	22
Apple Cinn Squares, Kellogg	23
Apple Jacks	26
Apple Raisin Crisp	25
Arrowhead Crunch	18
Arrowhead Mills Instant	23
Blueberry Squares, Kellogg's	23
Booberry	24
Bran Buds	22
Bran Chex	24
Bran Flakes	20
Cap'n Crunch	23
Cap'n Crunch's Cruchberries	24
Cap'n Crunch's Peanut Butter	22
Cheerios	20
Cheerios, Apple Cinnamon	22
Cheerios, Honey Nut	23
Cinnamon Life	19
Cinnamon Toast Crunch	22
Cocoa Crispies	25
Cocoa Pebbles	25
Cocoa Puffs	25

carbohydrates (grams)

* Counts are based on average-size servings (as indicated
on package) and without added milk.

11

CEREALS*, Part 2

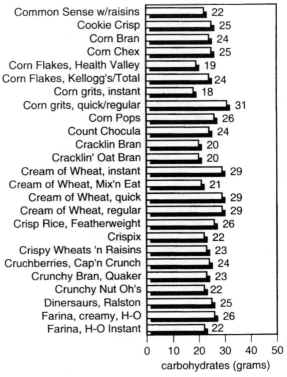

Cereal	carbohydrates (grams)
Common Sense w/raisins	22
Cookie Crisp	25
Corn Bran	24
Corn Chex	25
Corn Flakes, Health Valley	19
Corn Flakes, Kellogg's/Total	24
Corn grits, instant	18
Corn grits, quick/regular	31
Corn Pops	26
Count Chocula	24
Cracklin Bran	20
Cracklin' Oat Bran	20
Cream of Wheat, instant	29
Cream of Wheat, Mix'n Eat	21
Cream of Wheat, quick	29
Cream of Wheat, regular	29
Crisp Rice, Featherweight	26
Crispix	22
Crispy Wheats 'n Raisins	23
Cruchberries, Cap'n Crunch	24
Crunchy Bran, Quaker	23
Crunchy Nut Oh's	22
Dinersaurs, Ralston	25
Farina, creamy, H-O	26
Farina, H-O Instant	22

carbohydrates (grams)

* Counts are based on average-size servings (as indicated
on package) and without added milk.

12

CEREALS*, Part 3

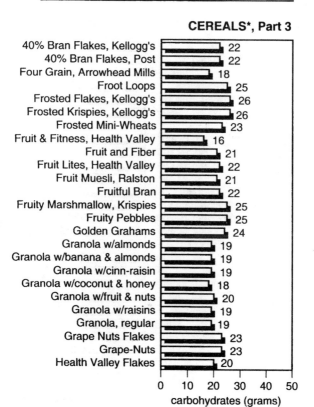

Cereal	carbohydrates (grams)
40% Bran Flakes, Kellogg's	22
40% Bran Flakes, Post	22
Four Grain, Arrowhead Mills	18
Froot Loops	25
Frosted Flakes, Kellogg's	26
Frosted Krispies, Kellogg's	26
Frosted Mini-Wheats	23
Fruit & Fitness, Health Valley	16
Fruit and Fiber	21
Fruit Lites, Health Valley	22
Fruit Muesli, Ralston	21
Fruitful Bran	22
Fruity Marshmallow, Krispies	25
Fruity Pebbles	25
Golden Grahams	24
Granola w/almonds	19
Granola w/banana & almonds	19
Granola w/cinn-raisin	19
Granola w/coconut & honey	18
Granola w/fruit & nuts	20
Granola w/raisins	19
Granola, regular	19
Grape Nuts Flakes	23
Grape-Nuts	23
Health Valley Flakes	20

carbohydrates (grams)

* Counts are based on average-size servings (as indicated on package) and without added milk.

CEREALS*, Part 4

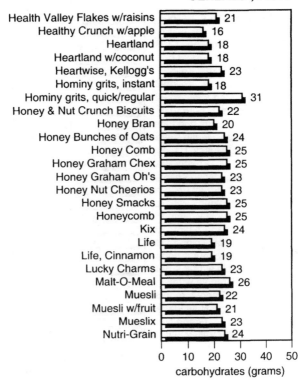

Cereal	carbohydrates (grams)
Health Valley Flakes w/raisins	21
Healthy Crunch w/apple	16
Heartland	18
Heartland w/coconut	18
Heartwise, Kellogg's	23
Hominy grits, instant	18
Hominy grits, quick/regular	31
Honey & Nut Crunch Biscuits	22
Honey Bran	20
Honey Bunches of Oats	24
Honey Comb	25
Honey Graham Chex	25
Honey Graham Oh's	23
Honey Nut Cheerios	23
Honey Smacks	25
Honeycomb	25
Kix	24
Life	19
Life, Cinnamon	19
Lucky Charms	23
Malt-O-Meal	26
Muesli	22
Muesli w/fruit	21
Mueslix	23
Nutri-Grain	24

carbohydrates (grams)

* Counts are based on average-size servings (as indicated
on package) and without added milk.

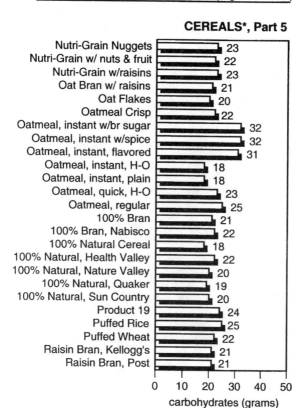

Alphabetical Chart
(for Hi-Low Comparison Charts, see pages 83 - 164)

CEREALS*, Part 5

Cereal	carbohydrates (grams)
Nutri-Grain Nuggets	23
Nutri-Grain w/ nuts & fruit	22
Nutri-Grain w/raisins	23
Oat Bran w/ raisins	21
Oat Flakes	20
Oatmeal Crisp	22
Oatmeal, instant w/br sugar	32
Oatmeal, instant w/spice	32
Oatmeal, instant, flavored	31
Oatmeal, instant, H-O	18
Oatmeal, instant, plain	18
Oatmeal, quick, H-O	23
Oatmeal, regular	25
100% Bran	21
100% Bran, Nabisco	22
100% Natural Cereal	18
100% Natural, Health Valley	22
100% Natural, Nature Valley	20
100% Natural, Quaker	19
100% Natural, Sun Country	20
Product 19	24
Puffed Rice	25
Puffed Wheat	22
Raisin Bran, Kellogg's	21
Raisin Bran, Post	21

carbohydrates (grams)

* Counts are based on average-size servings (as indicated on package) and without added milk.

CEREALS, Part 6

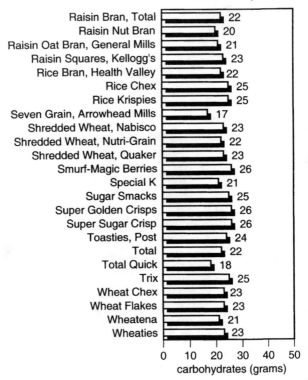

Cereal	carbohydrates (grams)
Raisin Bran, Total	22
Raisin Nut Bran	20
Raisin Oat Bran, General Mills	21
Raisin Squares, Kellogg's	23
Rice Bran, Health Valley	22
Rice Chex	25
Rice Krispies	25
Seven Grain, Arrowhead Mills	17
Shredded Wheat, Nabisco	23
Shredded Wheat, Nutri-Grain	22
Shredded Wheat, Quaker	23
Smurf-Magic Berries	26
Special K	21
Sugar Smacks	25
Super Golden Crisps	26
Super Sugar Crisp	26
Toasties, Post	24
Total	22
Total Quick	18
Trix	25
Wheat Chex	23
Wheat Flakes	23
Wheatena	21
Wheaties	23

* Counts are based on average-size servings (as indicated on package) and without added milk.

COMBINED AND FROZEN FOODS*,
Part 1

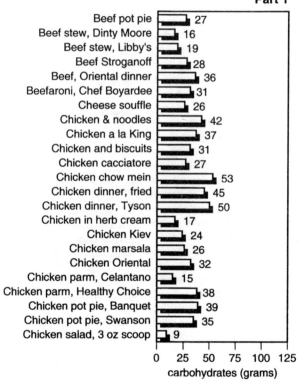

Food	carbohydrates (grams)
Beef pot pie	27
Beef stew, Dinty Moore	16
Beef stew, Libby's	19
Beef Stroganoff	28
Beef, Oriental dinner	36
Beefaroni, Chef Boyardee	31
Cheese souffle	26
Chicken & noodles	42
Chicken a la King	37
Chicken and biscuits	31
Chicken cacciatore	27
Chicken chow mein	53
Chicken dinner, fried	45
Chicken dinner, Tyson	50
Chicken in herb cream	17
Chicken Kiev	24
Chicken marsala	26
Chicken Oriental	32
Chicken parm, Celantano	15
Chicken parm, Healthy Choice	38
Chicken pot pie, Banquet	39
Chicken pot pie, Swanson	35
Chicken salad, 3 oz scoop	9

carbohydrates (grams)

* Counts are based on average-size servings as indicated
on package. Adjust count to reflect amount consumed.

COMBINED AND FROZEN FOODS*, Part 2

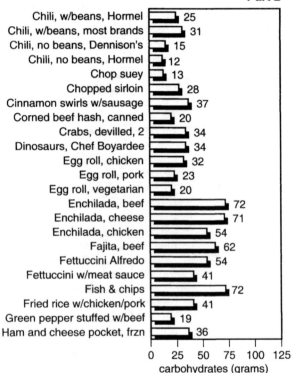

Food	carbohydrates (grams)
Chili, w/beans, Hormel	25
Chili, w/beans, most brands	31
Chili, no beans, Dennison's	15
Chili, no beans, Hormel	12
Chop suey	13
Chopped sirloin	28
Cinnamon swirls w/sausage	37
Corned beef hash, canned	20
Crabs, devilled, 2	34
Dinosaurs, Chef Boyardee	34
Egg roll, chicken	32
Egg roll, pork	23
Egg roll, vegetarian	20
Enchilada, beef	72
Enchilada, cheese	71
Enchilada, chicken	54
Fajita, beef	62
Fettuccini Alfredo	54
Fettuccini w/meat sauce	41
Fish & chips	72
Fried rice w/chicken/pork	41
Green pepper stuffed w/beef	19
Ham and cheese pocket, frzn	36

0   25   50   75   100   125
carbohydrates (grams)

* Counts are based on average-size servings as indicated
on package. Adjust count to reflect amount consumed.

COMBINED AND FROZEN FOODS*,
Part 3

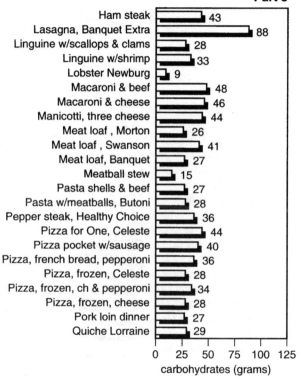

Food	carbohydrates (grams)
Ham steak	43
Lasagna, Banquet Extra	88
Linguine w/scallops & clams	28
Linguine w/shrimp	33
Lobster Newburg	9
Macaroni & beef	48
Macaroni & cheese	46
Manicotti, three cheese	44
Meat loaf , Morton	26
Meat loaf , Swanson	41
Meat loaf, Banquet	27
Meatball stew	15
Pasta shells & beef	27
Pasta w/meatballs, Butoni	28
Pepper steak, Healthy Choice	36
Pizza for One, Celeste	44
Pizza pocket w/sausage	40
Pizza, french bread, pepperoni	36
Pizza, frozen, Celeste	28
Pizza, frozen, ch & pepperoni	34
Pizza, frozen, cheese	28
Pork loin dinner	27
Quiche Lorraine	29

carbohydrates (grams)

* Counts are based on average-size servings as indicated
on package. Adjust count to reflect amount consumed.

COMBINED AND FROZEN FOODS*,
Part 4

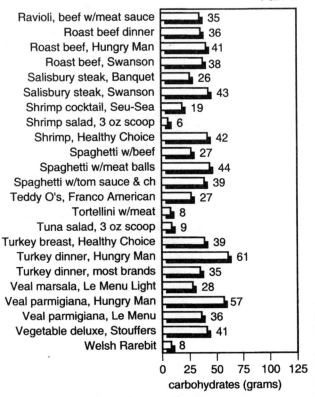

Food	carbohydrates (grams)
Ravioli, beef w/meat sauce	35
Roast beef dinner	36
Roast beef, Hungry Man	41
Roast beef, Swanson	38
Salisbury steak, Banquet	26
Salisbury steak, Swanson	43
Shrimp cocktail, Seu-Sea	19
Shrimp salad, 3 oz scoop	6
Shrimp, Healthy Choice	42
Spaghetti w/beef	27
Spaghetti w/meat balls	44
Spaghetti w/tom sauce & ch	39
Teddy O's, Franco American	27
Tortellini w/meat	8
Tuna salad, 3 oz scoop	9
Turkey breast, Healthy Choice	39
Turkey dinner, Hungry Man	61
Turkey dinner, most brands	35
Veal marsala, Le Menu Light	28
Veal parmigiana, Hungry Man	57
Veal parmigiana, Le Menu	36
Vegetable deluxe, Stouffers	41
Welsh Rarebit	8

carbohydrates (grams)

* Counts are based on average-size servings as indicated
on package. Adjust count to reflect amount consumed.

Dairy: CHEESE (HARD & SEMI-SOFT)*

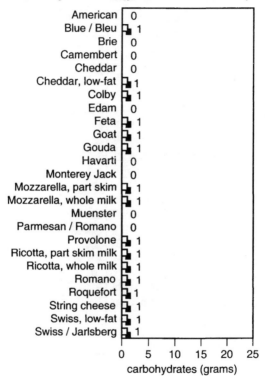

	carbohydrates (grams)
American	0
Blue / Bleu	1
Brie	0
Camembert	0
Cheddar	0
Cheddar, low-fat	1
Colby	1
Edam	0
Feta	1
Goat	1
Gouda	1
Havarti	0
Monterey Jack	0
Mozzarella, part skim	1
Mozzarella, whole milk	1
Muenster	0
Parmesan / Romano	0
Provolone	1
Ricotta, part skim milk	1
Ricotta, whole milk	1
Romano	1
Roquefort	1
String cheese	1
Swiss, low-fat	1
Swiss / Jarlsberg	1

0   5   10   15   20   25
carbohydrates (grams)

* Counts are based on one-ounce servings. Adjust count
to reflect amount consumed.

Dairy: CHEESES (SOFT), CREAMS & SUBSTITUTES*

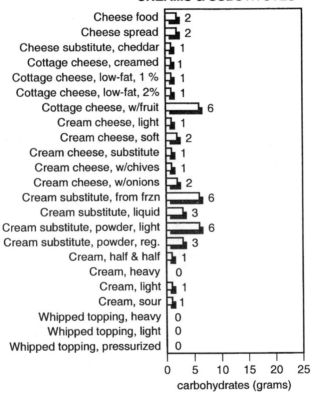

	carbohydrates (grams)
Cheese food	2
Cheese spread	2
Cheese substitute, cheddar	1
Cottage cheese, creamed	1
Cottage cheese, low-fat, 1 %	1
Cottage cheese, low-fat, 2%	1
Cottage cheese, w/fruit	6
Cream cheese, light	1
Cream cheese, soft	2
Cream cheese, substitute	1
Cream cheese, w/chives	1
Cream cheese, w/onions	2
Cream substitute, from frzn	6
Cream substitute, liquid	3
Cream substitute, powder, light	6
Cream substitute, powder, reg.	3
Cream, half & half	1
Cream, heavy	0
Cream, light	1
Cream, sour	1
Whipped topping, heavy	0
Whipped topping, light	0
Whipped topping, pressurized	0

carbohydrates (grams)

* Counts are based on one-ounce servings of soft cheese
or one tablespoon of cream or whipped topping.

Dairy: EGGS, MILK, YOGURT & SHAKES*

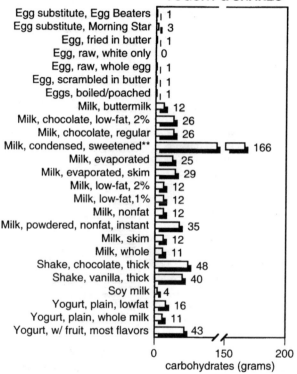

Item	carbohydrates (grams)
Egg substitute, Egg Beaters	1
Egg substitute, Morning Star	3
Egg, fried in butter	1
Egg, raw, white only	0
Egg, raw, whole egg	1
Egg, scrambled in butter	1
Eggs, boiled/poached	1
Milk, buttermilk	12
Milk, chocolate, low-fat, 2%	26
Milk, chocolate, regular	26
Milk, condensed, sweetened**	166
Milk, evaporated	25
Milk, evaporated, skim	29
Milk, low-fat, 2%	12
Milk, low-fat,1%	12
Milk, nonfat	12
Milk, powdered, nonfat, instant	35
Milk, skim	12
Milk, whole	11
Shake, chocolate, thick	48
Shake, vanilla, thick	40
Soy milk	4
Yogurt, plain, lowfat	16
Yogurt, plain, whole milk	11
Yogurt, w/ fruit, most flavors	43

0   150   200
carbohydrates (grams)

* Counts based on one egg or equivalent egg substitute or 8 fluid ounces of milk, yogurt, or shake.
** High count for this item requires break in bar.

23

Alphabetical Chart
(for Hi-Low Comparison Charts, see pages 83 - 164)

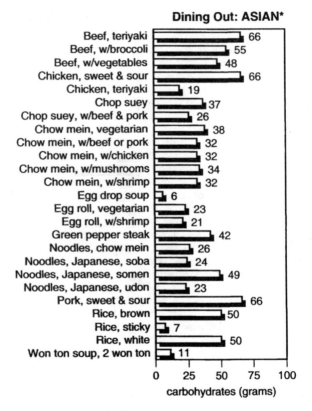

Dining Out: ASIAN*

Item	carbohydrates (grams)
Beef, teriyaki	66
Beef, w/broccoli	55
Beef, w/vegetables	48
Chicken, sweet & sour	66
Chicken, teriyaki	19
Chop suey	37
Chop suey, w/beef & pork	26
Chow mein, vegetarian	38
Chow mein, w/beef or pork	32
Chow mein, w/chicken	32
Chow mein, w/mushrooms	34
Chow mein, w/shrimp	32
Egg drop soup	6
Egg roll, vegetarian	23
Egg roll, w/shrimp	21
Green pepper steak	42
Noodles, chow mein	26
Noodles, Japanese, soba	24
Noodles, Japanese, somen	49
Noodles, Japanese, udon	23
Pork, sweet & sour	66
Rice, brown	50
Rice, sticky	7
Rice, white	50
Won ton soup, 2 won ton	11

carbohydrates (grams)

* Counts based on average-sized servings (for main dishes,
1 1/2 - 2 cups). Counts for main dishes include rice.

24

Dining Out: DELICATESSEN*

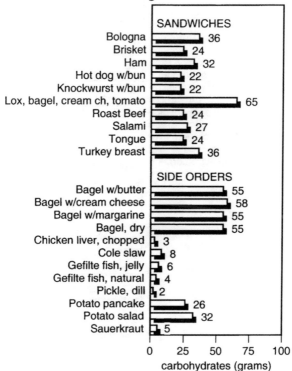

SANDWICHES

Bologna	36
Brisket	24
Ham	32
Hot dog w/bun	22
Knockwurst w/bun	22
Lox, bagel, cream ch, tomato	65
Roast Beef	24
Salami	27
Tongue	24
Turkey breast	36

SIDE ORDERS

Bagel w/butter	55
Bagel w/cream cheese	58
Bagel w/margarine	55
Bagel, dry	55
Chicken liver, chopped	3
Cole slaw	8
Gefilte fish, jelly	6
Gefilte fish, natural	4
Pickle, dill	2
Potato pancake	26
Potato salad	32
Sauerkraut	5

carbohydrates (grams)

* Unless otherwise indicated, counts based on average-
size servings or sandwiches. Sandwich counts assume
white or rye bread.

Dining Out: FRENCH AND OTHER INTERNATIONAL DISHES*

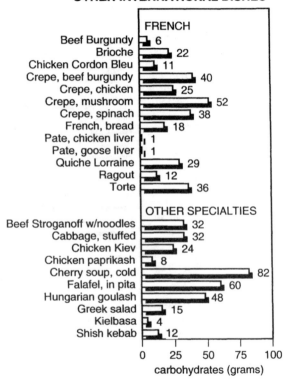

FRENCH

Dish	carbohydrates (grams)
Beef Burgundy	6
Brioche	22
Chicken Cordon Bleu	11
Crepe, beef burgundy	40
Crepe, chicken	25
Crepe, mushroom	52
Crepe, spinach	38
French, bread	18
Pate, chicken liver	1
Pate, goose liver	1
Quiche Lorraine	29
Ragout	12
Torte	36

OTHER SPECIALTIES

Dish	carbohydrates (grams)
Beef Stroganoff w/noodles	32
Cabbage, stuffed	32
Chicken Kiev	24
Chicken paprikash	8
Cherry soup, cold	82
Falafel, in pita	60
Hungarian goulash	48
Greek salad	15
Kielbasa	4
Shish kebab	12

carbohydrates (grams)

* Counts based on average-sized servings (for main dishes, 1 1/2 - 2 cups).

Alphabetical Chart
(for Hi-Low Comparison Charts, see pages 83 - 164)

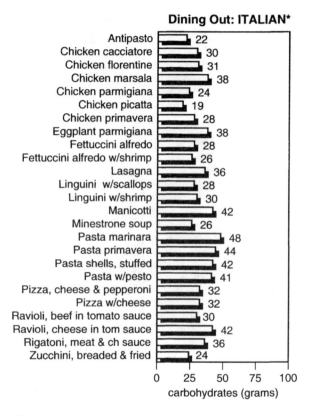

Dining Out: ITALIAN*

Food	carbohydrates (grams)
Antipasto	22
Chicken cacciatore	30
Chicken florentine	31
Chicken marsala	38
Chicken parmigiana	24
Chicken picatta	19
Chicken primavera	28
Eggplant parmigiana	38
Fettuccini alfredo	28
Fettuccini alfredo w/shrimp	26
Lasagna	36
Linguini w/scallops	28
Linguini w/shrimp	30
Manicotti	42
Minestrone soup	26
Pasta marinara	48
Pasta primavera	44
Pasta shells, stuffed	42
Pasta w/pesto	41
Pizza, cheese & pepperoni	32
Pizza w/cheese	32
Ravioli, beef in tomato sauce	30
Ravioli, cheese in tom sauce	42
Rigatoni, meat & ch sauce	36
Zucchini, breaded & fried	24

* Counts are based on average-sized servings (1 1/2 - 2 cups); for pizza, on 1/6 medium or 1/8 large pizza).

Dining Out: MEXICAN*

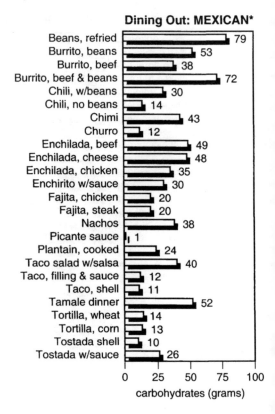

Food	carbohydrates (grams)
Beans, refried	79
Burrito, beans	53
Burrito, beef	38
Burrito, beef & beans	72
Chili, w/beans	30
Chili, no beans	14
Chimi	43
Churro	12
Enchilada, beef	49
Enchilada, cheese	48
Enchilada, chicken	35
Enchirito w/sauce	30
Fajita, chicken	20
Fajita, steak	20
Nachos	38
Picante sauce	1
Plantain, cooked	24
Taco salad w/salsa	40
Taco, filling & sauce	12
Taco, shell	11
Tamale dinner	52
Tortilla, wheat	14
Tortilla, corn	13
Tostada shell	10
Tostada w/sauce	26

carbohydrates (grams)

* Counts based on average-sized servings (for main dishes, 1 1/2 - 2 cups).

28

Fast Food: ARBY'S*

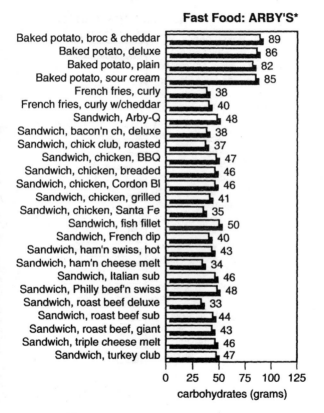

Item	carbohydrates (grams)
Baked potato, broc & cheddar	89
Baked potato, deluxe	86
Baked potato, plain	82
Baked potato, sour cream	85
French fries, curly	38
French fries, curly w/cheddar	40
Sandwich, Arby-Q	48
Sandwich, bacon'n ch, deluxe	38
Sandwich, chick club, roasted	37
Sandwich, chicken, BBQ	47
Sandwich, chicken, breaded	46
Sandwich, chicken, Cordon Bl	46
Sandwich, chicken, grilled	41
Sandwich, chicken, Santa Fe	35
Sandwich, fish fillet	50
Sandwich, French dip	40
Sandwich, ham'n swiss, hot	43
Sandwich, ham'n cheese melt	34
Sandwich, Italian sub	46
Sandwich, Philly beef'n swiss	48
Sandwich, roast beef deluxe	33
Sandwich, roast beef sub	44
Sandwich, roast beef, giant	43
Sandwich, triple cheese melt	46
Sandwich, turkey club	47

carbohydrates (grams)

* Unless otherwise indicated, counts are based on average-size servings.

Fast Food: BOSTON MARKET*

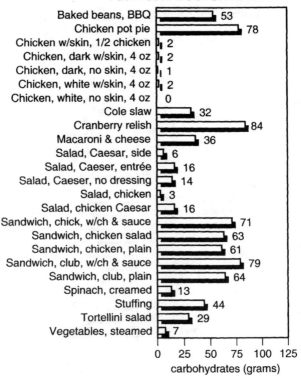

Item	carbohydrates (grams)
Baked beans, BBQ	53
Chicken pot pie	78
Chicken w/skin, 1/2 chicken	2
Chicken, dark w/skin, 4 oz	2
Chicken, dark, no skin, 4 oz	1
Chicken, white w/skin, 4 oz	2
Chicken, white, no skin, 4 oz	0
Cole slaw	32
Cranberry relish	84
Macaroni & cheese	36
Salad, Caesar, side	6
Salad, Caeser, entrée	16
Salad, Caeser, no dressing	14
Salad, chicken	3
Salad, chicken Caesar	16
Sandwich, chick, w/ch & sauce	71
Sandwich, chicken salad	63
Sandwich, chicken, plain	61
Sandwich, club, w/ch & sauce	79
Sandwich, club, plain	64
Spinach, creamed	13
Stuffing	44
Tortellini salad	29
Vegetables, steamed	7

carbohydrates (grams)

* Unless otherwise indicated, counts are based on average-size servings.

Fast Food: BURGER KING*

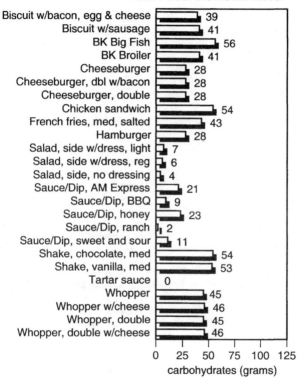

Item	carbohydrates (grams)
Biscuit w/bacon, egg & cheese	39
Biscuit w/sausage	41
BK Big Fish	56
BK Broiler	41
Cheeseburger	28
Cheeseburger, dbl w/bacon	28
Cheeseburger, double	28
Chicken sandwich	54
French fries, med, salted	43
Hamburger	28
Salad, side w/dress, light	7
Salad, side w/dress, reg	6
Salad, side, no dressing	4
Sauce/Dip, AM Express	21
Sauce/Dip, BBQ	9
Sauce/Dip, honey	23
Sauce/Dip, ranch	2
Sauce/Dip, sweet and sour	11
Shake, chocolate, med	54
Shake, vanilla, med	53
Tartar sauce	0
Whopper	45
Whopper w/cheese	46
Whopper, double	45
Whopper, double w/cheese	46

* Unless otherwise indicated, counts are based on average-size servings.

31

Fast Food: HARDEE'S*

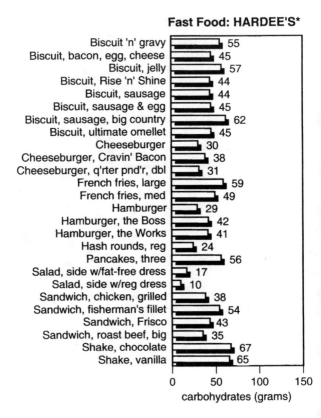

Item	carbohydrates (grams)
Biscuit 'n' gravy	55
Biscuit, bacon, egg, cheese	45
Biscuit, jelly	57
Biscuit, Rise 'n' Shine	44
Biscuit, sausage	44
Biscuit, sausage & egg	45
Biscuit, sausage, big country	62
Biscuit, ultimate omellet	45
Cheeseburger	30
Cheeseburger, Cravin' Bacon	38
Cheeseburger, q'rter pnd'r, dbl	31
French fries, large	59
French fries, med	49
Hamburger	29
Hamburger, the Boss	42
Hamburger, the Works	41
Hash rounds, reg	24
Pancakes, three	56
Salad, side w/fat-free dress	17
Salad, side w/reg dress	10
Sandwich, chicken, grilled	38
Sandwich, fisherman's fillet	54
Sandwich, Frisco	43
Sandwich, roast beef, big	35
Shake, chocolate	67
Shake, vanilla	65

carbohydrates (grams)

* Unless otherwise indicated, counts are based on average-size servings.

Fast Food: JACK IN THE BOX*

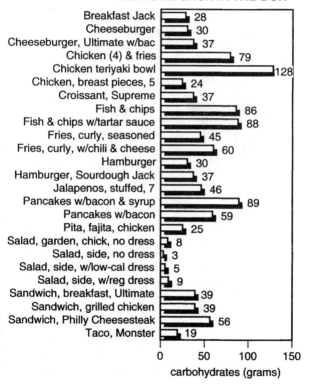

Item	carbohydrates (grams)
Breakfast Jack	28
Cheeseburger	30
Cheeseburger, Ultimate w/bac	37
Chicken (4) & fries	79
Chicken teriyaki bowl	128
Chicken, breast pieces, 5	24
Croissant, Supreme	37
Fish & chips	86
Fish & chips w/tartar sauce	88
Fries, curly, seasoned	45
Fries, curly, w/chili & cheese	60
Hamburger	30
Hamburger, Sourdough Jack	37
Jalapenos, stuffed, 7	46
Pancakes w/bacon & syrup	89
Pancakes w/bacon	59
Pita, fajita, chicken	25
Salad, garden, chick, no dress	8
Salad, side, no dress	3
Salad, side, w/low-cal dress	5
Salad, side, w/reg dress	9
Sandwich, breakfast, Ultimate	39
Sandwich, grilled chicken	39
Sandwich, Philly Cheesesteak	56
Taco, Monster	19

* Unless otherwise indicated, counts are based on average-size servings.

33

Fast Food: KFC*

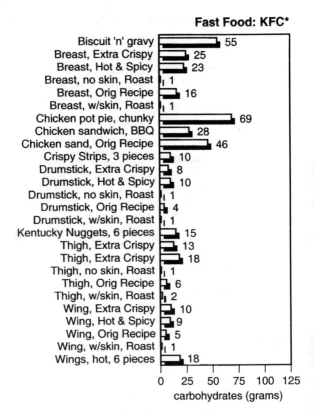

	carbohydrates (grams)
Biscuit 'n' gravy	55
Breast, Extra Crispy	25
Breast, Hot & Spicy	23
Breast, no skin, Roast	1
Breast, Orig Recipe	16
Breast, w/skin, Roast	1
Chicken pot pie, chunky	69
Chicken sandwich, BBQ	28
Chicken sand, Orig Recipe	46
Crispy Strips, 3 pieces	10
Drumstick, Extra Crispy	8
Drumstick, Hot & Spicy	10
Drumstick, no skin, Roast	1
Drumstick, Orig Recipe	4
Drumstick, w/skin, Roast	1
Kentucky Nuggets, 6 pieces	15
Thigh, Extra Crispy	13
Thigh, Extra Crispy	18
Thigh, no skin, Roast	1
Thigh, Orig Recipe	6
Thigh, w/skin, Roast	2
Wing, Extra Crispy	10
Wing, Hot & Spicy	9
Wing, Orig Recipe	5
Wing, w/skin, Roast	1
Wings, hot, 6 pieces	18

* Unless otherwise indicated, counts are based on average-size servings.

Alphabetical Chart
(for Hi-Low Comparison Charts, see pages 83 - 164)

Fast Food: MC DONALD'S*

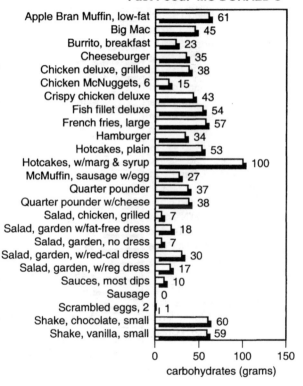

Item	carbohydrates (grams)
Apple Bran Muffin, low-fat	61
Big Mac	45
Burrito, breakfast	23
Cheeseburger	35
Chicken deluxe, grilled	38
Chicken McNuggets, 6	15
Crispy chicken deluxe	43
Fish fillet deluxe	54
French fries, large	57
Hamburger	34
Hotcakes, plain	53
Hotcakes, w/marg & syrup	100
McMuffin, sausage w/egg	27
Quarter pounder	37
Quarter pounder w/cheese	38
Salad, chicken, grilled	7
Salad, garden w/fat-free dress	18
Salad, garden, no dress	7
Salad, garden, w/red-cal dress	30
Salad, garden, w/reg dress	17
Sauces, most dips	10
Sausage	0
Scrambled eggs, 2	1
Shake, chocolate, small	60
Shake, vanilla, small	59

carbohydrates (grams)

* Unless otherwise indicated, counts are based on average-size servings.

Fast Food: PIZZA HUT*

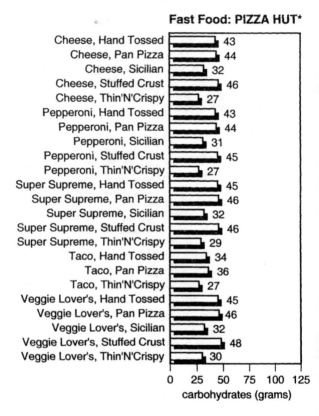

	carbohydrates (grams)
Cheese, Hand Tossed	43
Cheese, Pan Pizza	44
Cheese, Sicilian	32
Cheese, Stuffed Crust	46
Cheese, Thin'N'Crispy	27
Pepperoni, Hand Tossed	43
Pepperoni, Pan Pizza	44
Pepperoni, Sicilian	31
Pepperoni, Stuffed Crust	45
Pepperoni, Thin'N'Crispy	27
Super Supreme, Hand Tossed	45
Super Supreme, Pan Pizza	46
Super Supreme, Sicilian	32
Super Supreme, Stuffed Crust	46
Super Supreme, Thin'N'Crispy	29
Taco, Hand Tossed	34
Taco, Pan Pizza	36
Taco, Thin'N'Crispy	27
Veggie Lover's, Hand Tossed	45
Veggie Lover's, Pan Pizza	46
Veggie Lover's, Sicilian	32
Veggie Lover's, Stuffed Crust	48
Veggie Lover's, Thin'N'Crispy	30

0   25   50   75   100   125
carbohydrates (grams)

* Unless otherwise indicated, counts are based on average-size servings.

Alphabetical Chart
(for Hi-Low Comparison Charts, see pages 83 - 164)

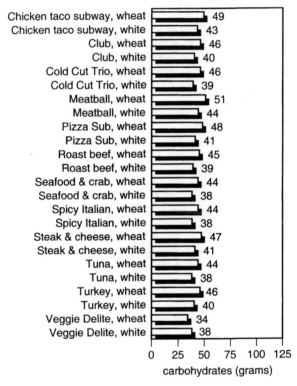

Fast Food: SUBWAY*

Item	carbohydrates (grams)
Chicken taco subway, wheat	49
Chicken taco subway, white	43
Club, wheat	46
Club, white	40
Cold Cut Trio, wheat	46
Cold Cut Trio, white	39
Meatball, wheat	51
Meatball, white	44
Pizza Sub, wheat	48
Pizza Sub, white	41
Roast beef, wheat	45
Roast beef, white	39
Seafood & crab, wheat	44
Seafood & crab, white	38
Spicy Italian, wheat	44
Spicy Italian, white	38
Steak & cheese, wheat	47
Steak & cheese, white	41
Tuna, wheat	44
Tuna, white	38
Turkey, wheat	46
Turkey, white	40
Veggie Delite, wheat	34
Veggie Delite, white	38

carbohydrates (grams)

* Unless otherwise indicated, counts are based on average-size servings.

37

Fast Food: TACO BELL*

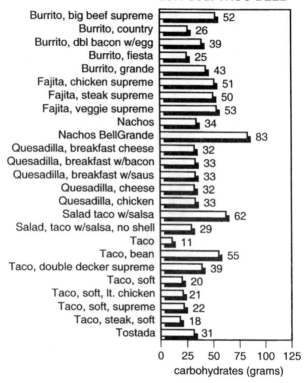

Item	carbohydrates (grams)
Burrito, big beef supreme	52
Burrito, country	26
Burrito, dbl bacon w/egg	39
Burrito, fiesta	25
Burrito, grande	43
Fajita, chicken supreme	51
Fajita, steak supreme	50
Fajita, veggie supreme	53
Nachos	34
Nachos BellGrande	83
Quesadilla, breakfast cheese	32
Quesadilla, breakfast w/bacon	33
Quesadilla, breakfast w/saus	33
Quesadilla, cheese	32
Quesadilla, chicken	33
Salad taco w/salsa	62
Salad, taco w/salsa, no shell	29
Taco	11
Taco, bean	55
Taco, double decker supreme	39
Taco, soft	20
Taco, soft, lt. chicken	21
Taco, soft, supreme	22
Taco, steak, soft	18
Tostada	31

* Unless otherwise indicated, counts are based on average-size servings.

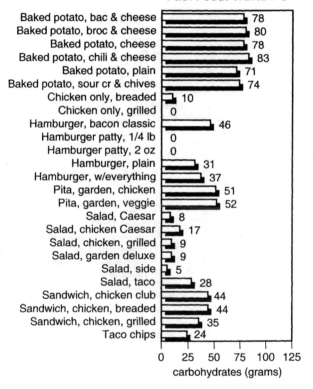

Fast Food: WENDY'S*

Item	carbohydrates (grams)
Baked potato, bac & cheese	78
Baked potato, broc & cheese	80
Baked potato, cheese	78
Baked potato, chili & cheese	83
Baked potato, plain	71
Baked potato, sour cr & chives	74
Chicken only, breaded	10
Chicken only, grilled	0
Hamburger, bacon classic	46
Hamburger patty, 1/4 lb	0
Hamburger patty, 2 oz	0
Hamburger, plain	31
Hamburger, w/everything	37
Pita, garden, chicken	51
Pita, garden, veggie	52
Salad, Caesar	8
Salad, chicken Caesar	17
Salad, chicken, grilled	9
Salad, garden deluxe	9
Salad, side	5
Salad, taco	28
Sandwich, chicken club	44
Sandwich, chicken, breaded	44
Sandwich, chicken, grilled	35
Taco chips	24

* Unless otherwise indicated, counts are based on average-size servings.

Fruits: FRESH & DRIED FRUITS AND JUICES *, Part 1

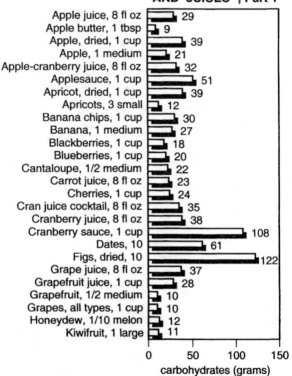

	carbohydrates (grams)
Apple juice, 8 fl oz	29
Apple butter, 1 tbsp	9
Apple, dried, 1 cup	39
Apple, 1 medium	21
Apple-cranberry juice, 8 fl oz	32
Applesauce, 1 cup	51
Apricot, dried, 1 cup	39
Apricots, 3 small	12
Banana chips, 1 cup	30
Banana, 1 medium	27
Blackberries, 1 cup	18
Blueberries, 1 cup	20
Cantaloupe, 1/2 medium	22
Carrot juice, 8 fl oz	23
Cherries, 1 cup	24
Cran juice cocktail, 8 fl oz	35
Cranberry juice, 8 fl oz	38
Cranberry sauce, 1 cup	108
Dates, 10	61
Figs, dried, 10	122
Grape juice, 8 fl oz	37
Grapefruit juice, 1 cup	28
Grapefruit, 1/2 medium	10
Grapes, all types, 1 cup	10
Honeydew, 1/10 melon	12
Kiwifruit, 1 large	11

0   50   100   150
carbohydrates (grams)

* Unless otherwise indicated, counts are based on one whole, fresh fruit.

Fruits: FRESH & DRIED FRUITS
AND JUICES *, Part 2

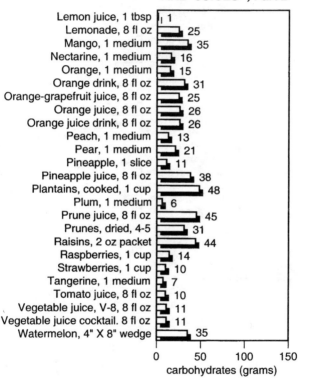

	carbohydrates (grams)
Lemon juice, 1 tbsp	1
Lemonade, 8 fl oz	25
Mango, 1 medium	35
Nectarine, 1 medium	16
Orange, 1 medium	15
Orange drink, 8 fl oz	31
Orange-grapefruit juice, 8 fl oz	25
Orange juice, 8 fl oz	26
Orange juice drink, 8 fl oz	26
Peach, 1 medium	13
Pear, 1 medium	21
Pineapple, 1 slice	11
Pineapple juice, 8 fl oz	38
Plantains, cooked, 1 cup	48
Plum, 1 medium	6
Prune juice, 8 fl oz	45
Prunes, dried, 4-5	31
Raisins, 2 oz packet	44
Raspberries, 1 cup	14
Strawberries, 1 cup	10
Tangerine, 1 medium	7
Tomato juice, 8 fl oz	10
Vegetable juice, V-8, 8 fl oz	11
Vegetable juice cocktail, 8 fl oz	11
Watermelon, 4" X 8" wedge	35

* Unless otherwise indicated, counts are based on one
  whole, fresh fruit.

41

GRAVIES, SAUCES & DIPS*

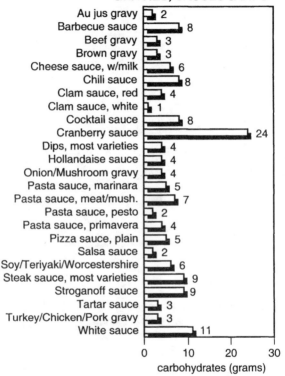

Food	carbohydrates (grams)
Au jus gravy	2
Barbecue sauce	8
Beef gravy	3
Brown gravy	3
Cheese sauce, w/milk	6
Chili sauce	8
Clam sauce, red	4
Clam sauce, white	1
Cocktail sauce	8
Cranberry sauce	24
Dips, most varieties	4
Hollandaise sauce	4
Onion/Mushroom gravy	4
Pasta sauce, marinara	5
Pasta sauce, meat/mush.	7
Pasta sauce, pesto	2
Pasta sauce, primavera	4
Pizza sauce, plain	5
Salsa sauce	2
Soy/Teriyaki/Worcestershire	6
Steak sauce, most varieties	9
Stroganoff sauce	9
Tartar sauce	3
Turkey/Chicken/Pork gravy	3
White sauce	11

* Counts are based on one-quarter cup servings.

MEATS*, Part 1

	BEEF
Bottom round, lean	0
Bottom round, regular	0
Brisket, lean	0
Brisket, regular	0
Chuck, blade, lean	0
Chuck, blade, regular	0
Corned beef	1
Ground beef, lean	0
Ground beef, regular	0
Rib roast, lean	0
Rib roast, regular	0
Short ribs, lean	0
Short ribs, regular	0
Steak, sirloin, lean	0
Steak, sirloin, regular	0
	LAMB
Chops, arm, lean	0
Chops, arm, regular	0
Chops, loin, lean	0
Chops, loin, regular	0
Leg, lean	0
Leg, lean, regular	0
Rack rib, lean	0
Rack rib, regular	0

0   5   10   15   20   25

carbohydrates (grams)

* Counts are based on 3-ounce servings.

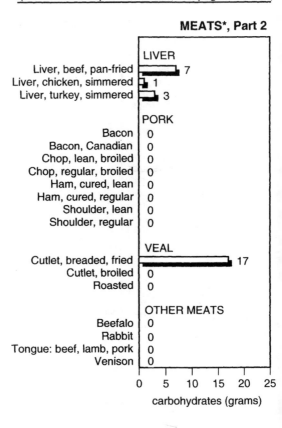

MEATS*, Part 2

LIVER
- Liver, beef, pan-fried — 7
- Liver, chicken, simmered — 1
- Liver, turkey, simmered — 3

PORK
- Bacon — 0
- Bacon, Canadian — 0
- Chop, lean, broiled — 0
- Chop, regular, broiled — 0
- Ham, cured, lean — 0
- Ham, cured, regular — 0
- Shoulder, lean — 0
- Shoulder, regular — 0

VEAL
- Cutlet, breaded, fried — 17
- Cutlet, broiled — 0
- Roasted — 0

OTHER MEATS
- Beefalo — 0
- Rabbit — 0
- Tongue: beef, lamb, pork — 0
- Venison — 0

carbohydrates (grams)

* Counts are based on 3-ounce servings.

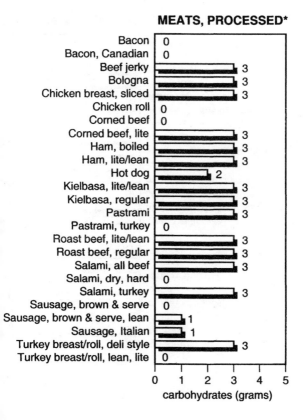

MEATS, PROCESSED*

Item	carbohydrates (grams)
Bacon	0
Bacon, Canadian	0
Beef jerky	3
Bologna	3
Chicken breast, sliced	3
Chicken roll	0
Corned beef	0
Corned beef, lite	3
Ham, boiled	3
Ham, lite/lean	3
Hot dog	2
Kielbasa, lite/lean	3
Kielbasa, regular	3
Pastrami	3
Pastrami, turkey	0
Roast beef, lite/lean	3
Roast beef, regular	3
Salami, all beef	3
Salami, dry, hard	0
Salami, turkey	3
Sausage, brown & serve	0
Sausage, brown & serve, lean	1
Sausage, Italian	1
Turkey breast/roll, deli style	3
Turkey breast/roll, lean, lite	0

* Counts are based on 3-ounce servings.

45

Medications: COUGH DROPS & SYRUPS*

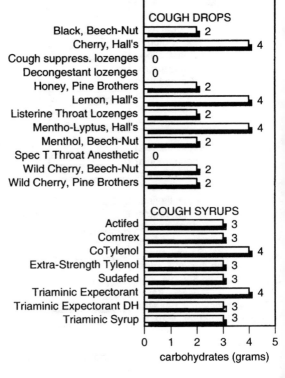

COUGH DROPS

Black, Beech-Nut	2
Cherry, Hall's	4
Cough suppress. lozenges	0
Decongestant lozenges	0
Honey, Pine Brothers	2
Lemon, Hall's	4
Listerine Throat Lozenges	2
Mentho-Lyptus, Hall's	4
Menthol, Beech-Nut	2
Spec T Throat Anesthetic	0
Wild Cherry, Beech-Nut	2
Wild Cherry, Pine Brothers	2

COUGH SYRUPS

Actifed	3
Comtrex	3
CoTylenol	4
Extra-Strength Tylenol	3
Sudafed	3
Triaminic Expectorant	4
Triaminic Expectorant DH	3
Triaminic Syrup	3

carbohydrates (grams)

* Counts are based on one cough drop or on recommende
doses for adults.

46

Medications: OVER-THE-COUNTER REMEDIES & VITAMINS AND MINERALS*

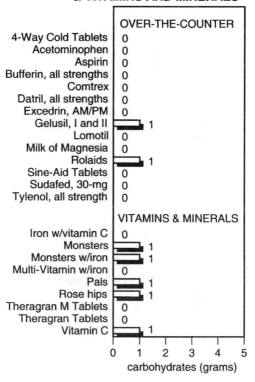

	carbohydrates (grams)
OVER-THE-COUNTER	
4-Way Cold Tablets	0
Acetaminophen	0
Aspirin	0
Bufferin, all strengths	0
Comtrex	0
Datril, all strengths	0
Excedrin, AM/PM	0
Gelusil, I and II	1
Lomotil	0
Milk of Magnesia	0
Rolaids	1
Sine-Aid Tablets	0
Sudafed, 30-mg	0
Tylenol, all strength	0
VITAMINS & MINERALS	
Iron w/vitamin C	0
Monsters	1
Monsters w/iron	1
Multi-Vitamin w/iron	0
Pals	1
Rose hips	1
Theragran M Tablets	0
Theragran Tablets	0
Vitamin C	1

carbohydrates (grams)

* Counts are based on recommended doses for adults.

MISCELLANEOUS FOODS*

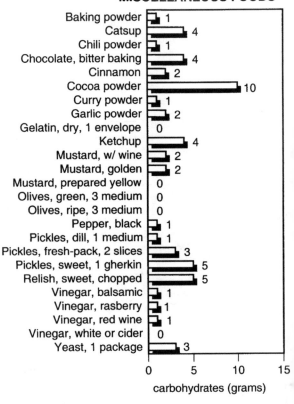

Food	carbohydrates (grams)
Baking powder	1
Catsup	4
Chili powder	1
Chocolate, bitter baking	4
Cinnamon	2
Cocoa powder	10
Curry powder	1
Garlic powder	2
Gelatin, dry, 1 envelope	0
Ketchup	4
Mustard, w/ wine	2
Mustard, golden	2
Mustard, prepared yellow	0
Olives, green, 3 medium	0
Olives, ripe, 3 medium	0
Pepper, black	1
Pickles, dill, 1 medium	1
Pickles, fresh-pack, 2 slices	3
Pickles, sweet, 1 gherkin	5
Relish, sweet, chopped	5
Vinegar, balsamic	1
Vinegar, rasberry	1
Vinegar, red wine	1
Vinegar, white or cider	0
Yeast, 1 package	3

carbohydrates (grams)

* Unless otherwise indicated, counts are based on a
one-tablespoon serving.

NUTS, BEANS AND SEEDS*: Part 1

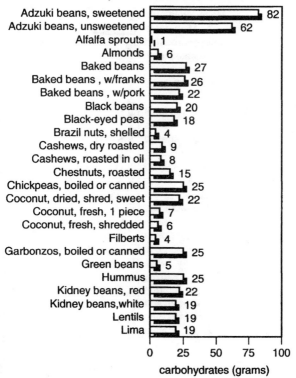

	carbohydrates (grams)
Adzuki beans, sweetened	82
Adzuki beans, unsweetened	62
Alfalfa sprouts	1
Almonds	6
Baked beans	27
Baked beans , w/franks	26
Baked beans , w/pork	22
Black beans	20
Black-eyed peas	18
Brazil nuts, shelled	4
Cashews, dry roasted	9
Cashews, roasted in oil	8
Chestnuts, roasted	15
Chickpeas, boiled or canned	25
Coconut, dried, shred, sweet	22
Coconut, fresh, 1 piece	7
Coconut, fresh, shredded	6
Filberts	4
Garbonzos, boiled or canned	25
Green beans	5
Hummus	25
Kidney beans, red	22
Kidney beans,white	19
Lentils	19
Lima	19

carbohydrates (grams)

* Unless otherwise indicated, counts are based on 1/2 cup
tofu or cooked beans or one-ounce servings of raw nuts or
seeds.

NUTS, BEANS AND SEEDS*: Part 2

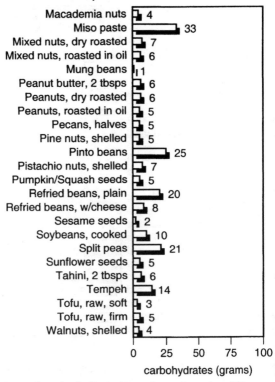

	carbohydrates (grams)
Macadamia nuts	4
Miso paste	33
Mixed nuts, dry roasted	7
Mixed nuts, roasted in oil	6
Mung beans	1
Peanut butter, 2 tbsps	6
Peanuts, dry roasted	6
Peanuts, roasted in oil	5
Pecans, halves	5
Pine nuts, shelled	5
Pinto beans	25
Pistachio nuts, shelled	7
Pumpkin/Squash seeds	5
Refried beans, plain	20
Refried beans, w/cheese	8
Sesame seeds	2
Soybeans, cooked	10
Split peas	21
Sunflower seeds	5
Tahini, 2 tbsps	6
Tempeh	14
Tofu, raw, soft	3
Tofu, raw, firm	5
Walnuts, shelled	4

carbohydrates (grams)

* Unless otherwise indicated, counts are based on 1/2 cup
tofu or cooked beans or one-ounce servings of raw nuts or
seeds.

50

OILS AND FATS*

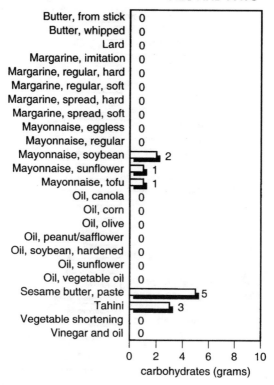

	carbohydrates (grams)
Butter, from stick	0
Butter, whipped	0
Lard	0
Margarine, imitation	0
Margarine, regular, hard	0
Margarine, regular, soft	0
Margarine, spread, hard	0
Margarine, spread, soft	0
Mayonnaise, eggless	0
Mayonnaise, regular	0
Mayonnaise, soybean	2
Mayonnaise, sunflower	1
Mayonnaise, tofu	1
Oil, canola	0
Oil, corn	0
Oil, olive	0
Oil, peanut/safflower	0
Oil, soybean, hardened	0
Oil, sunflower	0
Oil, vegetable oil	0
Sesame butter, paste	5
Tahini	3
Vegetable shortening	0
Vinegar and oil	0

* Counts are based on 1-tablespoon servings.

PASTA, WHOLE GRAINS, RICE & NOODLES*, Part 1

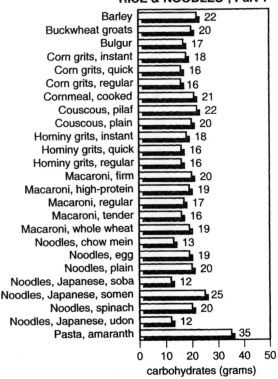

Food	carbohydrates (grams)
Barley	22
Buckwheat groats	20
Bulgur	17
Corn grits, instant	18
Corn grits, quick	16
Corn grits, regular	16
Cornmeal, cooked	21
Couscous, pilaf	22
Couscous, plain	20
Hominy grits, instant	18
Hominy grits, quick	16
Hominy grits, regular	16
Macaroni, firm	20
Macaroni, high-protein	19
Macaroni, regular	17
Macaroni, tender	16
Macaroni, whole wheat	19
Noodles, chow mein	13
Noodles, egg	19
Noodles, plain	20
Noodles, Japanese, soba	12
Noodles, Japanese, somen	25
Noodles, spinach	20
Noodles, Japanese, udon	12
Pasta, amaranth	35

carbohydrates (grams)

* Counts are based on cooked, 1/2-cup servings.

PASTA, WHOLE GRAINS, RICE & NOODLES*, Part 2

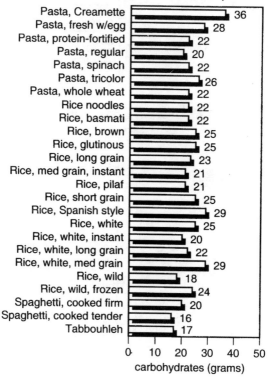

Food	carbohydrates (grams)
Pasta, Creamette	36
Pasta, fresh w/egg	28
Pasta, protein-fortified	22
Pasta, regular	20
Pasta, spinach	22
Pasta, tricolor	26
Pasta, whole wheat	22
Rice noodles	22
Rice, basmati	22
Rice, brown	25
Rice, glutinous	25
Rice, long grain	23
Rice, med grain, instant	21
Rice, pilaf	21
Rice, short grain	25
Rice, Spanish style	29
Rice, white	25
Rice, white, instant	20
Rice, white, long grain	22
Rice, white, med grain	29
Rice, wild	18
Rice, wild, frozen	24
Spaghetti, cooked firm	20
Spaghetti, cooked tender	16
Tabbouhleh	17

carbohydrates (grams)

* Counts are based on cooked, 1/2-cup servings.

Poultry: CHICKEN, TURKEY, AND OTHER FOWL*

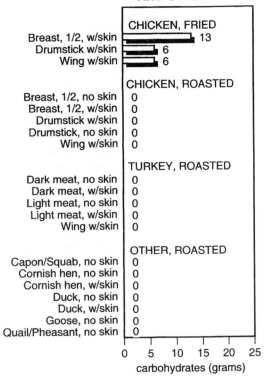

CHICKEN, FRIED
Breast, 1/2, w/skin — 13
Drumstick w/skin — 6
Wing w/skin — 6

CHICKEN, ROASTED
Breast, 1/2, no skin — 0
Breast, 1/2, w/skin — 0
Drumstick w/skin — 0
Drumstick, no skin — 0
Wing w/skin — 0

TURKEY, ROASTED
Dark meat, no skin — 0
Dark meat, w/skin — 0
Light meat, no skin — 0
Light meat, w/skin — 0
Wing w/skin — 0

OTHER, ROASTED
Capon/Squab, no skin — 0
Cornish hen, no skin — 0
Cornish hen, w/skin — 0
Duck, no skin — 0
Duck, w/skin — 0
Goose, no skin — 0
Quail/Pheasant, no skin — 0

carbohydrates (grams)
0   5   10   15   20   25

* Unless otherwise indicated, counts are based on 3-ounce
servings.

SALAD BAR CHOICES*

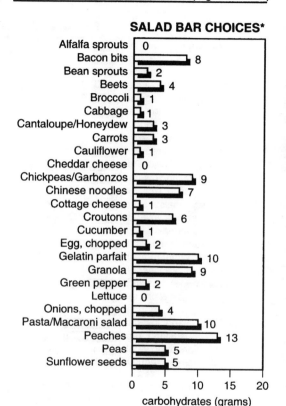

Salad Bar Choice	carbohydrates (grams)
Alfalfa sprouts	0
Bacon bits	8
Bean sprouts	2
Beets	4
Broccoli	1
Cabbage	1
Cantaloupe/Honeydew	3
Carrots	3
Cauliflower	1
Cheddar cheese	0
Chickpeas/Garbonzos	9
Chinese noodles	7
Cottage cheese	1
Croutons	6
Cucumber	1
Egg, chopped	2
Gelatin parfait	10
Granola	9
Green pepper	2
Lettuce	0
Onions, chopped	4
Pasta/Macaroni salad	10
Peaches	13
Peas	5
Sunflower seeds	5

carbohydrates (grams)

* Counts are based on one-quarter cup servings.

55

SALAD DRESSING*

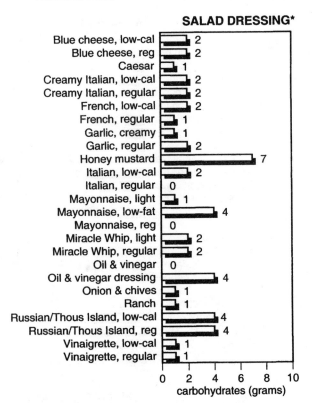

Dressing	carbohydrates (grams)
Blue cheese, low-cal	2
Blue cheese, reg	2
Caesar	1
Creamy Italian, low-cal	2
Creamy Italian, regular	2
French, low-cal	2
French, regular	1
Garlic, creamy	1
Garlic, regular	2
Honey mustard	7
Italian, low-cal	2
Italian, regular	0
Mayonnaise, light	1
Mayonnaise, low-fat	4
Mayonnaise, reg	0
Miracle Whip, light	2
Miracle Whip, regular	2
Oil & vinegar	0
Oil & vinegar dressing	4
Onion & chives	1
Ranch	1
Russian/Thous Island, low-cal	4
Russian/Thous Island, reg	4
Vinaigrette, low-cal	1
Vinaigrette, regular	1

* For ease of comparison, counts are based on single tablespoon servings. Adjust counts to reflect quantities consumed.

SEAFOOD*, Part 1

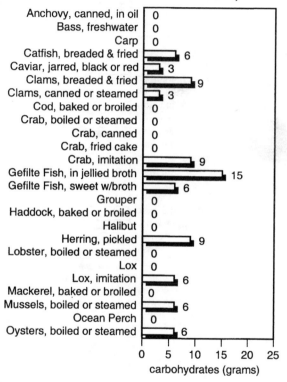

Food	carbohydrates (grams)
Anchovy, canned, in oil	0
Bass, freshwater	0
Carp	0
Catfish, breaded & fried	6
Caviar, jarred, black or red	3
Clams, breaded & fried	9
Clams, canned or steamed	3
Cod, baked or broiled	0
Crab, boiled or steamed	0
Crab, canned	0
Crab, fried cake	0
Crab, imitation	9
Gefilte Fish, in jellied broth	15
Gefilte Fish, sweet w/broth	6
Grouper	0
Haddock, baked or broiled	0
Halibut	0
Herring, pickled	9
Lobster, boiled or steamed	0
Lox	0
Lox, imitation	6
Mackerel, baked or broiled	0
Mussels, boiled or steamed	6
Ocean Perch	0
Oysters, boiled or steamed	6

carbohydrates (grams)

* Counts are based on 3-ounce servings. Canned seafood items are assumed to be drained.

SEAFOOD*, Part 2

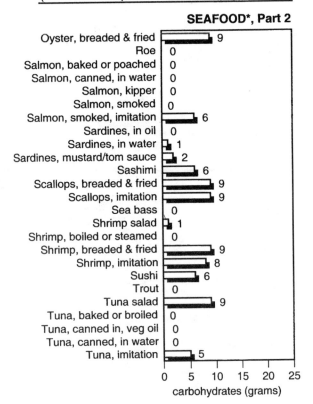

Item	carbohydrates (grams)
Oyster, breaded & fried	9
Roe	0
Salmon, baked or poached	0
Salmon, canned, in water	0
Salmon, kipper	0
Salmon, smoked	0
Salmon, smoked, imitation	6
Sardines, in oil	0
Sardines, in water	1
Sardines, mustard/tom sauce	2
Sashimi	6
Scallops, breaded & fried	9
Scallops, imitation	9
Sea bass	0
Shrimp salad	1
Shrimp, boiled or steamed	0
Shrimp, breaded & fried	9
Shrimp, imitation	8
Sushi	6
Trout	0
Tuna salad	9
Tuna, baked or broiled	0
Tuna, canned in, veg oil	0
Tuna, canned, in water	0
Tuna, imitation	5

carbohydrates (grams)

* Counts are based on 3-ounce servings. Canned seafood
items are assumed to be drained.

SNACK FOODS AND CHIPS*: Part 1

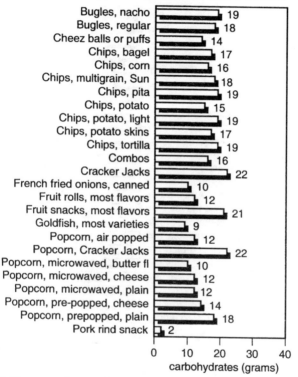

	carbohydrates (grams)
Bugles, nacho	19
Bugles, regular	18
Cheez balls or puffs	14
Chips, bagel	17
Chips, corn	16
Chips, multigrain, Sun	18
Chips, pita	19
Chips, potato	15
Chips, potato, light	19
Chips, potato skins	17
Chips, tortilla	19
Combos	16
Cracker Jacks	22
French fried onions, canned	10
Fruit rolls, most flavors	12
Fruit snacks, most flavors	21
Goldfish, most varieties	9
Popcorn, air popped	12
Popcorn, Cracker Jacks	22
Popcorn, microwaved, butter fl	10
Popcorn, microwaved, cheese	12
Popcorn, microwaved, plain	12
Popcorn, pre-popped, cheese	14
Popcorn, prepopped, plain	18
Pork rind snack	2

* For ease of comparison, counts are based on one-ounce
servings. For popcorn, 1 ounce unpopped = 2 cups popped.
Adjust count to reflect amount consumed.

SNACK FOODS AND CHIPS*: Part 2

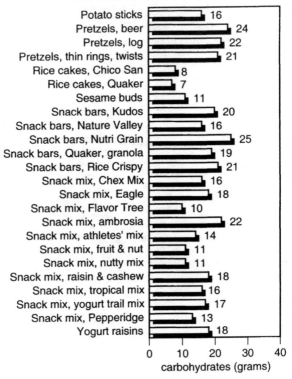

	carbohydrates (grams)
Potato sticks	16
Pretzels, beer	24
Pretzels, log	22
Pretzels, thin rings, twists	21
Rice cakes, Chico San	8
Rice cakes, Quaker	7
Sesame buds	11
Snack bars, Kudos	20
Snack bars, Nature Valley	16
Snack bars, Nutri Grain	25
Snack bars, Quaker, granola	19
Snack bars, Rice Crispy	21
Snack mix, Chex Mix	16
Snack mix, Eagle	18
Snack mix, Flavor Tree	10
Snack mix, ambrosia	22
Snack mix, athletes' mix	14
Snack mix, fruit & nut	11
Snack mix, nutty mix	11
Snack mix, raisin & cashew	18
Snack mix, tropical mix	16
Snack mix, yogurt trail mix	17
Snack mix, Pepperidge	13
Yogurt raisins	18

* For ease of comparison, counts are based on one-ounce
servings. For popcorn, 1 ounce unpopped = 2 cups popped.
Adjust count to reflect amount consumed.

SOUP*: Part 1

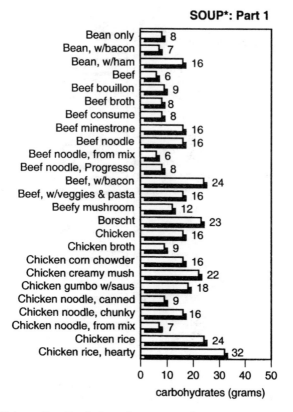

Soup	carbohydrates (grams)
Bean only	8
Bean, w/bacon	7
Bean, w/ham	16
Beef	6
Beef bouillon	9
Beef broth	8
Beef consume	8
Beef minestrone	16
Beef noodle	16
Beef noodle, from mix	6
Beef noodle, Progresso	8
Beef, w/bacon	24
Beef, w/veggies & pasta	16
Beefy mushroom	12
Borscht	23
Chicken	16
Chicken broth	9
Chicken corn chowder	16
Chicken creamy mush	22
Chicken gumbo w/saus	18
Chicken noodle, canned	9
Chicken noodle, chunky	16
Chicken noodle, from mix	7
Chicken rice	24
Chicken rice, hearty	32

carbohydrates (grams)

* Unless otherwise indicated, counts are based on one-cup servings.

Alphabetical Chart
(for Hi-Low Comparison Charts, see pages 83 - 164)

SOUP*, Part 2

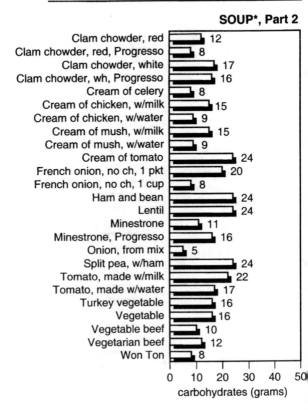

Soup	carbohydrates (grams)
Clam chowder, red	12
Clam chowder, red, Progresso	8
Clam chowder, white	17
Clam chowder, wh, Progresso	16
Cream of celery	8
Cream of chicken, w/milk	15
Cream of chicken, w/water	9
Cream of mush, w/milk	15
Cream of mush, w/water	9
Cream of tomato	24
French onion, no ch, 1 pkt	20
French onion, no ch, 1 cup	8
Ham and bean	24
Lentil	24
Minestrone	11
Minestrone, Progresso	16
Onion, from mix	5
Split pea, w/ham	24
Tomato, made w/milk	22
Tomato, made w/water	17
Turkey vegetable	16
Vegetable	16
Vegetable beef	10
Vegetarian beef	12
Won Ton	8

carbohydrates (grams) — 0, 10, 20, 30, 40, 50

* Unless otherwise indicated, counts are based on one-cup servings.

Sweets: CAKES*, Part 1

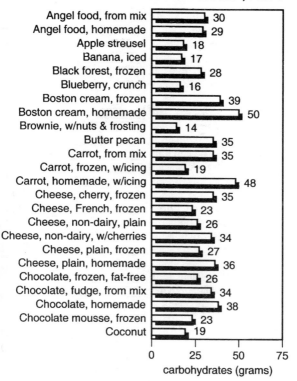

Cake	carbohydrates (grams)
Angel food, from mix	30
Angel food, homemade	29
Apple streusel	18
Banana, iced	17
Black forest, frozen	28
Blueberry, crunch	16
Boston cream, frozen	39
Boston cream, homemade	50
Brownie, w/nuts & frosting	14
Butter pecan	35
Carrot, from mix	35
Carrot, frozen, w/icing	19
Carrot, homemade, w/icing	48
Cheese, cherry, frozen	35
Cheese, French, frozen	23
Cheese, non-dairy, plain	26
Cheese, non-dairy, w/cherries	34
Cheese, plain, frozen	27
Cheese, plain, homemade	36
Chocolate, frozen, fat-free	26
Chocolate, fudge, from mix	34
Chocolate, homemade	38
Chocolate mousse, frozen	23
Coconut	19

carbohydrates (grams)

* Counts are based on average-size pieces and slices,
  where appropriate, as indicated on package.

63

Sweets: CAKES*, Part 2

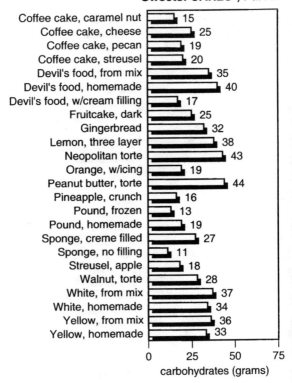

Cake	carbohydrates (grams)
Coffee cake, caramel nut	15
Coffee cake, cheese	25
Coffee cake, pecan	19
Coffee cake, streusel	20
Devil's food, from mix	35
Devil's food, homemade	40
Devil's food, w/cream filling	17
Fruitcake, dark	25
Gingerbread	32
Lemon, three layer	38
Neopolitan torte	43
Orange, w/icing	19
Peanut butter, torte	44
Pineapple, crunch	16
Pound, frozen	13
Pound, homemade	19
Sponge, creme filled	27
Sponge, no filling	11
Streusel, apple	18
Walnut, torte	28
White, from mix	37
White, homemade	34
Yellow, from mix	36
Yellow, homemade	33

carbohydrates (grams)

* Counts are based on average-size pieces and slices,
where appropriate, as indicated on package.

Alphabetical Chart
(for Hi-Low Comparison Charts, see pages 83 - 164)

Sweets: SNACK CAKES*

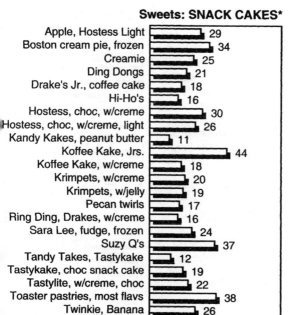

Item	carbohydrate (grams)
Apple, Hostess Light	29
Boston cream pie, frozen	34
Creamie	25
Ding Dongs	21
Drake's Jr., coffee cake	18
Hi-Ho's	16
Hostess, choc, w/creme	30
Hostess, choc, w/creme, light	26
Kandy Kakes, peanut butter	11
Koffee Kake, Jrs.	44
Koffee Kake, w/creme	18
Krimpets, w/creme	20
Krimpets, w/jelly	19
Pecan twirls	17
Ring Ding, Drakes, w/creme	16
Sara Lee, fudge, frozen	24
Suzy Q's	37
Tandy Takes, Tastykake	12
Tastykake, choc snack cake	19
Tastylite, w/creme, choc	22
Toaster pastries, most flavs	38
Twinkie, Banana	26
Twinkies, Fruit N Creme	27
Twinkies, w/creme	27
Twinkies, w/creme, light	21

carbohydrate (grams)

* Counts based on serving size as indicated on package.

Sweets: CANDY*, Part 1

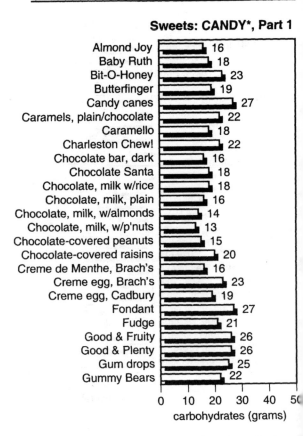

	carbohydrates (grams)
Almond Joy	16
Baby Ruth	18
Bit-O-Honey	23
Butterfinger	19
Candy canes	27
Caramels, plain/chocolate	22
Caramello	18
Charleston Chew!	22
Chocolate bar, dark	16
Chocolate Santa	18
Chocolate, milk w/rice	18
Chocolate, milk, plain	16
Chocolate, milk, w/almonds	14
Chocolate, milk, w/p'nuts	13
Chocolate-covered peanuts	15
Chocolate-covered raisins	20
Creme de Menthe, Brach's	16
Creme egg, Brach's	23
Creme egg, Cadbury	19
Fondant	27
Fudge	21
Good & Fruity	26
Good & Plenty	26
Gum drops	25
Gummy Bears	22

* For ease of comparison, counts are based on one-ounce servings. Adjust counts to reflect quantities consumed.

Sweets: CANDY*, Part 2

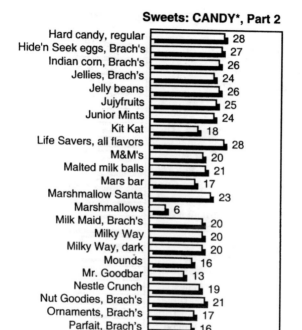

	carbohydrates (grams)
Hard candy, regular	28
Hide'n Seek eggs, Brach's	27
Indian corn, Brach's	26
Jellies, Brach's	24
Jelly beans	26
Jujyfruits	25
Junior Mints	24
Kit Kat	18
Life Savers, all flavors	28
M&M's	20
Malted milk balls	21
Mars bar	17
Marshmallow Santa	23
Marshmallows	6
Milk Maid, Brach's	20
Milky Way	20
Milky Way, dark	20
Mounds	16
Mr. Goodbar	13
Nestle Crunch	19
Nut Goodies, Brach's	21
Ornaments, Brach's	17
Parfait, Brach's	16
Peanut brittle	20
Peppermint Patties, York	23

* For ease of comparison, counts are based on one-ounce
servings. Adjust counts to reflect quantities consumed.

Sweets: CANDY*, Part 3

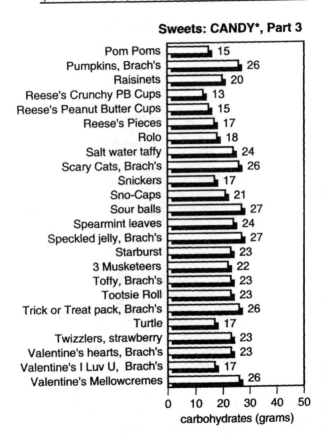

Candy	carbohydrates (grams)
Pom Poms	15
Pumpkins, Brach's	26
Raisinets	20
Reese's Crunchy PB Cups	13
Reese's Peanut Butter Cups	15
Reese's Pieces	17
Rolo	18
Salt water taffy	24
Scary Cats, Brach's	26
Snickers	17
Sno-Caps	21
Sour balls	27
Spearmint leaves	24
Speckled jelly, Brach's	27
Starburst	23
3 Musketeers	22
Toffy, Brach's	23
Tootsie Roll	23
Trick or Treat pack, Brach's	26
Turtle	17
Twizzlers, strawberry	23
Valentine's hearts, Brach's	23
Valentine's I Luv U, Brach's	17
Valentine's Mellowcremes	26

carbohydrates (grams)

* For ease of comparison, counts are based on one-ounce
servings. Adjust counts to reflect quantities consumed.

Sweets: COOKIES*, Part 1

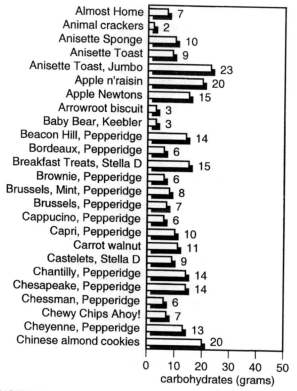

	carbohydrates (grams)
Almost Home	7
Animal crackers	2
Anisette Sponge	10
Anisette Toast	9
Anisette Toast, Jumbo	23
Apple n'raisin	20
Apple Newtons	15
Arrowroot biscuit	3
Baby Bear, Keebler	3
Beacon Hill, Pepperidge	14
Bordeaux, Pepperidge	6
Breakfast Treats, Stella D	15
Brownie, Pepperidge	6
Brussels, Mint, Pepperidge	8
Brussels, Pepperidge	7
Cappucino, Pepperidge	6
Capri, Pepperidge	10
Carrot walnut	11
Castelets, Stella D	9
Chantilly, Pepperidge	14
Chesapeake, Pepperidge	14
Chessman, Pepperidge	6
Chewy Chips Ahoy!	7
Cheyenne, Pepperidge	13
Chinese almond cookies	20

* NOTE: For ease of comparison, counts are based on
single cookie servings. When more than one cookie is
consumed, counts should be adjusted accordingly.

Sweets: COOKIES*, Part 2

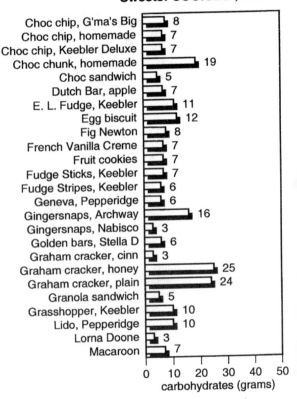

Cookie	carbohydrates (grams)
Choc chip, G'ma's Big	8
Choc chip, homemade	7
Choc chip, Keebler Deluxe	7
Choc chunk, homemade	19
Choc sandwich	5
Dutch Bar, apple	7
E. L. Fudge, Keebler	11
Egg biscuit	12
Fig Newton	8
French Vanilla Creme	7
Fruit cookies	7
Fudge Sticks, Keebler	7
Fudge Stripes, Keebler	6
Geneva, Pepperidge	6
Gingersnaps, Archway	16
Gingersnaps, Nabisco	3
Golden bars, Stella D	6
Graham cracker, cinn	3
Graham cracker, honey	25
Graham cracker, plain	24
Granola sandwich	5
Grasshopper, Keebler	10
Lido, Pepperidge	10
Lorna Doone	3
Macaroon	7

carbohydrates (grams)

* NOTE: For ease of comparison, counts are based on
single cookie servings. When more than one cookie is
consumed, counts should be adjusted accordingly.

Sweets: COOKIES*, Part 3

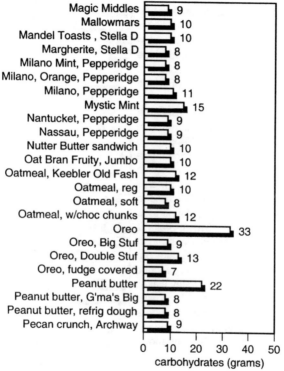

Cookie	carbohydrates (grams)
Magic Middles	9
Mallowmars	10
Mandel Toasts , Stella D	10
Margherite, Stella D	8
Milano Mint, Pepperidge	8
Milano, Orange, Pepperidge	8
Milano, Pepperidge	11
Mystic Mint	15
Nantucket, Pepperidge	9
Nassau, Pepperidge	9
Nutter Butter sandwich	10
Oat Bran Fruity, Jumbo	10
Oatmeal, Keebler Old Fash	12
Oatmeal, reg	10
Oatmeal, soft	8
Oatmeal, w/choc chunks	12
Oreo	33
Oreo, Big Stuf	9
Oreo, Double Stuf	13
Oreo, fudge covered	7
Peanut butter	22
Peanut butter, G'ma's Big	8
Peanut butter, refrig dough	8
Pecan crunch, Archway	9

carbohydrates (grams)

* NOTE: For ease of comparison, counts are based on
single cookie servings. When more than one cookie is
consumed, counts should be adjusted accordingly.

Sweets: COOKIES*, Part 4

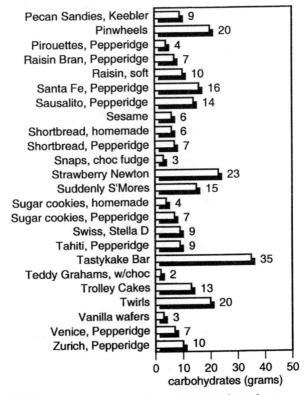

	carbohydrates (grams)
Pecan Sandies, Keebler	9
Pinwheels	20
Pirouettes, Pepperidge	4
Raisin Bran, Pepperidge	7
Raisin, soft	10
Santa Fe, Pepperidge	16
Sausalito, Pepperidge	14
Sesame	6
Shortbread, homemade	6
Shortbread, Pepperidge	7
Snaps, choc fudge	3
Strawberry Newton	23
Suddenly S'Mores	15
Sugar cookies, homemade	4
Sugar cookies, Pepperidge	7
Swiss, Stella D	9
Tahiti, Pepperidge	9
Tastykake Bar	35
Teddy Grahams, w/choc	2
Trolley Cakes	13
Twirls	20
Vanilla wafers	3
Venice, Pepperidge	7
Zurich, Pepperidge	10

* NOTE: For ease of comparison, counts are based on
single cookie servings. When more than one cookie is
consumed, counts should be adjusted accordingly.

Sweets: DONUTS*

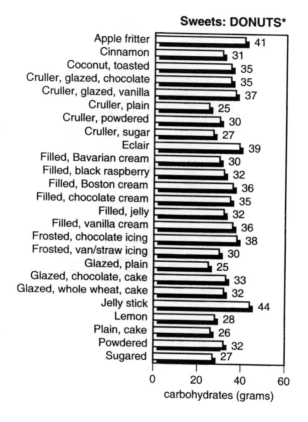

Donut	carbohydrates (grams)
Apple fritter	41
Cinnamon	31
Coconut, toasted	35
Cruller, glazed, chocolate	35
Cruller, glazed, vanilla	37
Cruller, plain	25
Cruller, powdered	30
Cruller, sugar	27
Eclair	39
Filled, Bavarian cream	30
Filled, black raspberry	32
Filled, Boston cream	36
Filled, chocolate cream	35
Filled, jelly	32
Filled, vanilla cream	36
Frosted, chocolate icing	38
Frosted, van/straw icing	30
Glazed, plain	25
Glazed, chocolate, cake	33
Glazed, whole wheat, cake	32
Jelly stick	44
Lemon	28
Plain, cake	26
Powdered	32
Sugared	27

carbohydrates (grams)

* Counts are based on average-size donuts.

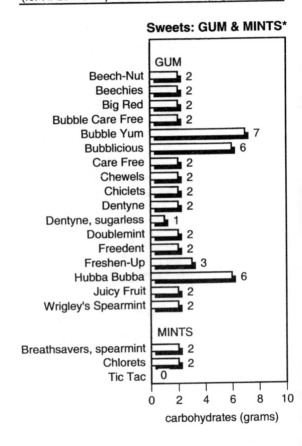

Sweets: GUM & MINTS*

GUM

Beech-Nut	2
Beechies	2
Big Red	2
Bubble Care Free	2
Bubble Yum	7
Bubblicious	6
Care Free	2
Chewels	2
Chiclets	2
Dentyne	2
Dentyne, sugarless	1
Doublemint	2
Freedent	2
Freshen-Up	3
Hubba Bubba	6
Juicy Fruit	2
Wrigley's Spearmint	2

MINTS

Breathsavers, spearmint	2
Chlorets	2
Tic Tac	0

carbohydrates (grams)

* Counts are based on single sticks or mints.

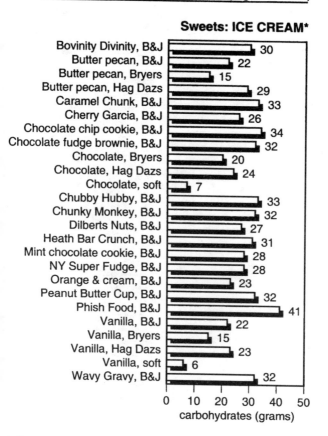

Sweets: ICE CREAM*

	carbohydrates (grams)
Bovinity Divinity, B&J	30
Butter pecan, B&J	22
Butter pecan, Bryers	15
Butter pecan, Hag Dazs	29
Caramel Chunk, B&J	33
Cherry Garcia, B&J	26
Chocolate chip cookie, B&J	34
Chocolate fudge brownie, B&J	32
Chocolate, Bryers	20
Chocolate, Hag Dazs	24
Chocolate, soft	7
Chubby Hubby, B&J	33
Chunky Monkey, B&J	32
Dilberts Nuts, B&J	27
Heath Bar Crunch, B&J	31
Mint chocolate cookie, B&J	28
NY Super Fudge, B&J	28
Orange & cream, B&J	23
Peanut Butter Cup, B&J	32
Phish Food, B&J	41
Vanilla, B&J	22
Vanilla, Bryers	15
Vanilla, Hag Dazs	23
Vanilla, soft	6
Wavy Gravy, B&J	32

* Counts are based on one-half cup servings. "B&J"
  designates Ben & Jerry's brand.

Sweets: ICE CREAM CONES & BARS, ICE CREAM ALTERNATIVES AND PUDDINGS*

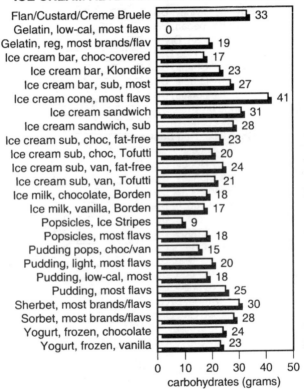

Food	carbohydrates (grams)
Flan/Custard/Creme Bruele	33
Gelatin, low-cal, most flavs	0
Gelatin, reg, most brands/flav	19
Ice cream bar, choc-covered	17
Ice cream bar, Klondike	23
Ice cream bar, sub, most	27
Ice cream cone, most flavs	41
Ice cream sandwich	31
Ice cream sandwich, sub	28
Ice cream sub, choc, fat-free	23
Ice cream sub, choc, Tofutti	20
Ice cream sub, van, fat-free	24
Ice cream sub, van, Tofutti	21
Ice milk, chocolate, Borden	18
Ice milk, vanilla, Borden	17
Popsicles, Ice Stripes	9
Popsicles, most flavs	18
Pudding pops, choc/van	15
Pudding, light, most flavs	20
Pudding, low-cal, most	18
Pudding, most flavs	25
Sherbet, most brands/flavs	30
Sorbet, most brands/flavs	28
Yogurt, frozen, chocolate	24
Yogurt, frozen, vanilla	23

* Counts are based on average- or one-half cup servings.
"Sub" designates non-dairy, ice cream substitute.

Alphabetical Chart
(for Hi-Low Comparison Charts, see pages 83 - 164)

Sweets: PIES*

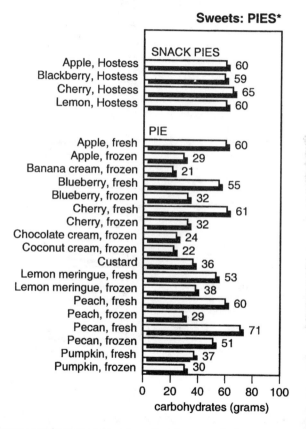

SNACK PIES

Apple, Hostess	60
Blackberry, Hostess	59
Cherry, Hostess	65
Lemon, Hostess	60

PIE

Apple, fresh	60
Apple, frozen	29
Banana cream, frozen	21
Blueberry, fresh	55
Blueberry, frozen	32
Cherry, fresh	61
Cherry, frozen	32
Chocolate cream, frozen	24
Coconut cream, frozen	22
Custard	36
Lemon meringue, fresh	53
Lemon meringue, frozen	38
Peach, fresh	60
Peach, frozen	29
Pecan, fresh	71
Pecan, frozen	51
Pumpkin, fresh	37
Pumpkin, frozen	30

0   20   40   60   80   100
carbohydrates (grams)

* Counts are based on average-size pieces and slices,
  where appropriate, as indicated on package.

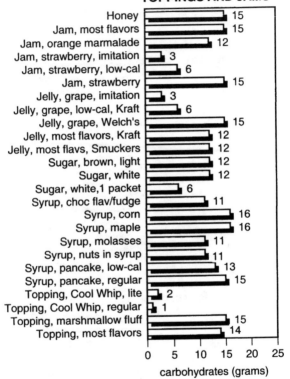

Alphabetical Chart
(for Hi-Low Comparison Charts, see pages 83 - 164)

Sweets: SUGARS, SYRUPS, TOPPINGS AND JAMS*

Item	carbohydrates (grams)
Honey	15
Jam, most flavors	15
Jam, orange marmalade	12
Jam, strawberry, imitation	3
Jam, strawberry, low-cal	6
Jam, strawberry	15
Jelly, grape, imitation	3
Jelly, grape, low-cal, Kraft	6
Jelly, grape, Welch's	15
Jelly, most flavors, Kraft	12
Jelly, most flavs, Smuckers	12
Sugar, brown, light	12
Sugar, white	12
Sugar, white, 1 packet	6
Syrup, choc flav/fudge	11
Syrup, corn	16
Syrup, maple	16
Syrup, molasses	11
Syrup, nuts in syrup	11
Syrup, pancake, low-cal	13
Syrup, pancake, regular	15
Topping, Cool Whip, lite	2
Topping, Cool Whip, regular	1
Topping, marshmallow fluff	15
Topping, most flavors	14

carbohydrates (grams)

* Counts are based on single-tablespoon servings. Jams and preserves can be assumed to have equal values.

78

VEGETABLES*, Part 1

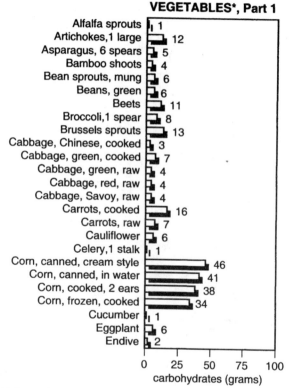

Vegetable	carbohydrates (grams)
Alfalfa sprouts	1
Artichokes, 1 large	12
Asparagus, 6 spears	5
Bamboo shoots	4
Bean sprouts, mung	6
Beans, green	6
Beets	11
Broccoli, 1 spear	8
Brussels sprouts	13
Cabbage, Chinese, cooked	3
Cabbage, green, cooked	7
Cabbage, green, raw	4
Cabbage, red, raw	4
Cabbage, Savoy, raw	4
Carrots, cooked	16
Carrots, raw	7
Cauliflower	6
Celery, 1 stalk	1
Corn, canned, cream style	46
Corn, canned, in water	41
Corn, cooked, 2 ears	38
Corn, frozen, cooked	34
Cucumber	1
Eggplant	6
Endive	2

carbohydrates (grams)
0   25   50   75   100

* Unless otherwise indicated, counts are based on one-cup servings. For vegetable juices, see the Fruits & Juices section.

VEGETABLES*, Part 2

Vegetable	carbohydrates (grams)
Greens	7
Kale	7
Kohlrabi, stems	11
Lettuce, Boston, 1/4 head	1
Lettuce, Cos, 1/4 head	2
Lettuce, Iceberg, 1/4 head	3
Lettuce, Romaine, 1/4 head	1
Mung bean, sprouted	6
Mushrooms, boiled/canned	8
Mushrooms, raw	3
Okra pods, 3 pods	2
Onions , cooked	13
Onions , raw	12
Parsnips	30
Pea pods, Chinese, cooked	11
Peas, green	22
Peppers, green, raw	4
Peppers, hot chili, 6	4
Peppers, red, raw	4
Plantain, cooked & sliced	48
Potato , au gratin	30
Potato salad	28
Potato, baked, 1 medium	51
Potato, french fries, baked, 14	24
Potato, french fries, 14	28

carbohydrates (grams)
0   25   50   75   100

* Unless otherwise indicated, counts are based on one-cup
servings. For vegetable juices, see the Fruits & Juices
section.

VEGETABLES*, Part 3

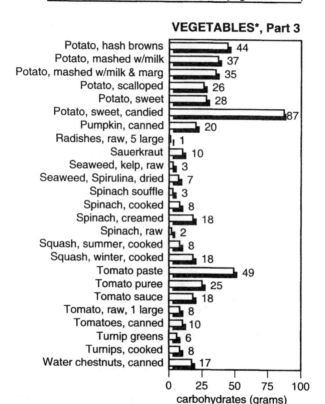

Vegetable	carbohydrates (grams)
Potato, hash browns	44
Potato, mashed w/milk	37
Potato, mashed w/milk & marg	35
Potato, scalloped	26
Potato, sweet	28
Potato, sweet, candied	87
Pumpkin, canned	20
Radishes, raw, 5 large	1
Sauerkraut	10
Seaweed, kelp, raw	3
Seaweed, Spirulina, dried	7
Spinach souffle	3
Spinach, cooked	8
Spinach, creamed	18
Spinach, raw	2
Squash, summer, cooked	8
Squash, winter, cooked	18
Tomato paste	49
Tomato puree	25
Tomato sauce	18
Tomato, raw, 1 large	8
Tomatoes, canned	10
Turnip greens	6
Turnips, cooked	8
Water chestnuts, canned	17

carbohydrates (grams)

* Unless otherwise indicated, counts are based on one-cup
servings. For vegetable juices, see the Fruits & Juices
section.

VEGETARIAN CHOICES*

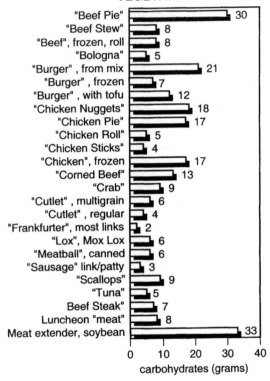

Item	carbohydrates (grams)
"Beef Pie"	30
"Beef Stew"	8
"Beef", frozen, roll	8
"Bologna"	5
"Burger", from mix	21
"Burger", frozen	7
"Burger", with tofu	12
"Chicken Nuggets"	18
"Chicken Pie"	17
"Chicken Roll"	5
"Chicken Sticks"	4
"Chicken", frozen	17
"Corned Beef"	13
"Crab"	9
"Cutlet", multigrain	6
"Cutlet", regular	4
"Frankfurter", most links	2
"Lox", Mox Lox	6
"Meatball", canned	6
"Sausage" link/patty	3
"Scallops"	9
"Tuna"	5
Beef Steak"	7
Luncheon "meat"	8
Meat extender, soybean	33

carbohydrates (grams)

* Made from tofu, textured vegetable protein or a combination of both. Counts are based on 3-ounce servings.

HI-LOW COMPARISON CHARTS

BEVERAGES*, Part 1

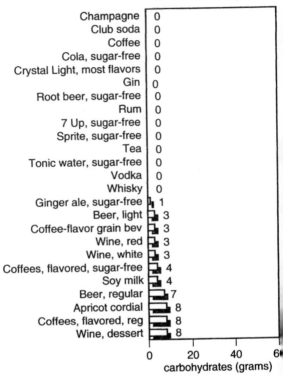

	carbohydrates (grams)
Champagne	0
Club soda	0
Coffee	0
Cola, sugar-free	0
Crystal Light, most flavors	0
Gin	0
Root beer, sugar-free	0
Rum	0
7 Up, sugar-free	0
Sprite, sugar-free	0
Tea	0
Tonic water, sugar-free	0
Vodka	0
Whisky	0
Ginger ale, sugar-free	1
Beer, light	3
Coffee-flavor grain bev	3
Wine, red	3
Wine, white	3
Coffees, flavored, sugar-free	4
Soy milk	4
Beer, regular	7
Apricot cordial	8
Coffees, flavored, reg	8
Wine, dessert	8

0   20   40   60

carbohydrates (grams)

* Counts for non-alcoholic drinks and beer are based on
8-fluid-ounce servings, for wine on 3 1/2-fluid-ounce
servings and, for hard liquor, on 1 1/2-fluid-ounce serving

BEVERAGES*, Part 2

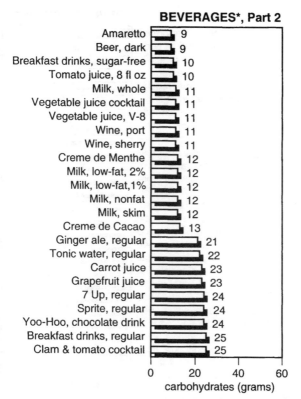

Beverage	carbohydrates (grams)
Amaretto	9
Beer, dark	9
Breakfast drinks, sugar-free	10
Tomato juice, 8 fl oz	10
Milk, whole	11
Vegetable juice cocktail	11
Vegetable juice, V-8	11
Wine, port	11
Wine, sherry	11
Creme de Menthe	12
Milk, low-fat, 2%	12
Milk, low-fat, 1%	12
Milk, nonfat	12
Milk, skim	12
Creme de Cacao	13
Ginger ale, regular	21
Tonic water, regular	22
Carrot juice	23
Grapefruit juice	23
7 Up, regular	24
Sprite, regular	24
Yoo-Hoo, chocolate drink	24
Breakfast drinks, regular	25
Clam & tomato cocktail	25

carbohydrates (grams)

* Counts for non-alcoholic drinks and beer are based on
8-fluid-ounce servings, for wine on 3 1/2-fluid-ounce
servings and, for hard liquor, on 1 1/2-fluid-ounce servings.

BEVERAGES*, Part 3

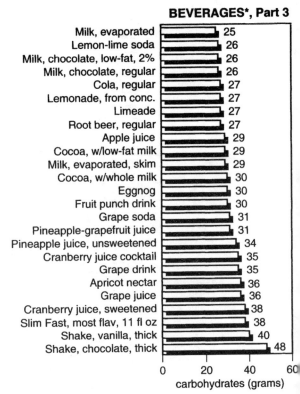

Beverage	carbohydrates (grams)
Milk, evaporated	25
Lemon-lime soda	26
Milk, chocolate, low-fat, 2%	26
Milk, chocolate, regular	26
Cola, regular	27
Lemonade, from conc.	27
Limeade	27
Root beer, regular	27
Apple juice	29
Cocoa, w/low-fat milk	29
Milk, evaporated, skim	29
Cocoa, w/whole milk	30
Eggnog	30
Fruit punch drink	30
Grape soda	31
Pineapple-grapefruit juice	31
Pineapple juice, unsweetened	34
Cranberry juice cocktail	35
Grape drink	35
Apricot nectar	36
Grape juice	36
Cranberry juice, sweetened	38
Slim Fast, most flav, 11 fl oz	38
Shake, vanilla, thick	40
Shake, chocolate, thick	48

carbohydrates (grams)

* Counts for non-alcoholic drinks and beer are based on
8-fluid-ounce servings, for wine on 3 1/2-fluid-ounce
servings and, for hard liquor, on 1 1/2-fluid-ounce servings

Bread, Crackers, and Flours:
BAGELS*

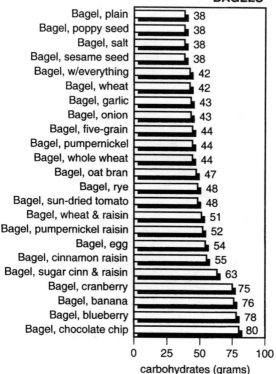

	carbohydrates (grams)
Bagel, plain	38
Bagel, poppy seed	38
Bagel, salt	38
Bagel, sesame seed	38
Bagel, w/everything	42
Bagel, wheat	42
Bagel, garlic	43
Bagel, onion	43
Bagel, five-grain	44
Bagel, pumpernickel	44
Bagel, whole wheat	44
Bagel, oat bran	47
Bagel, rye	48
Bagel, sun-dried tomato	48
Bagel, wheat & raisin	51
Bagel, pumpernickel raisin	52
Bagel, egg	54
Bagel, cinnamon raisin	55
Bagel, sugar cinn & raisin	63
Bagel, cranberry	75
Bagel, banana	76
Bagel, blueberry	78
Bagel, chocolate chip	80

Per one bagel, approximate weight: 3 ounces.

87

Bread, Crackers, and Flours:
BISCUITS, ROLLS & MUFFINS*

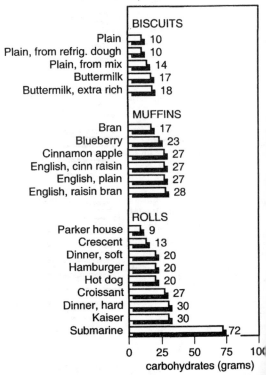

BISCUITS
Plain — 10
Plain, from refrig. dough — 10
Plain, from mix — 14
Buttermilk — 17
Buttermilk, extra rich — 18

MUFFINS
Bran — 17
Blueberry — 23
Cinnamon apple — 27
English, cinn raisin — 27
English, plain — 27
English, raisin bran — 28

ROLLS
Parker house — 9
Crescent — 13
Dinner, soft — 20
Hamburger — 20
Hot dog — 20
Croissant — 27
Dinner, hard — 30
Kaiser — 30
Submarine — 72

0   25   50   75   100
carbohydrates (grams)

* Counts are based on single, average-size items. Average
sweet muffin is assumed to be 2 3/4 inches by 2 inches.
Average sweet and English muffin weight is 57 grams.

Bread. Crackers, and Flours:
BREAD*

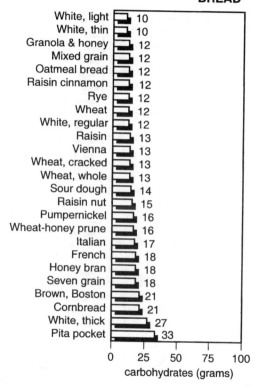

White, light	10
White, thin	10
Granola & honey	12
Mixed grain	12
Oatmeal bread	12
Raisin cinnamon	12
Rye	12
Wheat	12
White, regular	12
Raisin	13
Vienna	13
Wheat, cracked	13
Wheat, whole	13
Sour dough	14
Raisin nut	15
Pumpernickel	16
Wheat-honey prune	16
Italian	17
French	18
Honey bran	18
Seven grain	18
Brown, Boston	21
Cornbread	21
White, thick	27
Pita pocket	33

0   25   50   75   100
carbohydrates (grams)

* Counts are based on one single, average-size slice.

89

Bread, Crackers, and Flours:
CRACKERS*

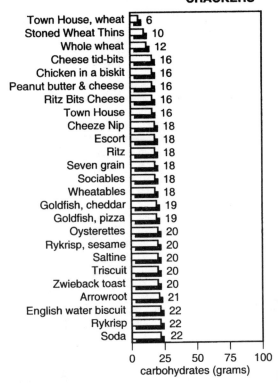

Cracker	carbohydrates (grams)
Town House, wheat	6
Stoned Wheat Thins	10
Whole wheat	12
Cheese tid-bits	16
Chicken in a biskit	16
Peanut butter & cheese	16
Ritz Bits Cheese	16
Town House	16
Cheeze Nip	18
Escort	18
Ritz	18
Seven grain	18
Sociables	18
Wheatables	18
Goldfish, cheddar	19
Goldfish, pizza	19
Oysterettes	20
Rykrisp, sesame	20
Saltine	20
Triscuit	20
Zwieback toast	20
Arrowroot	21
English water biscuit	22
Rykrisp	22
Soda	22

carbohydrates (grams)

* For ease of comparison, counts are based on one-ounce
servings. Adjust counts to reflect quantities consumed.

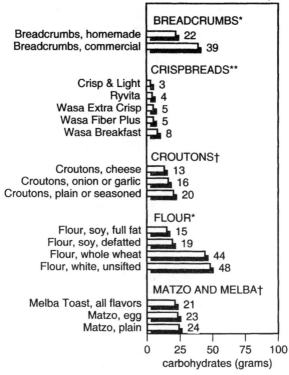

Hi-Low Comparison Chart
(for Alphabetical Charts, see pages 1 - 82)

**Bread, Crackers, and Flours:
DRY & CRISPY***

BREADCRUMBS*
Breadcrumbs, homemade — 22
Breadcrumbs, commercial — 39

CRISPBREADS**
Crisp & Light — 3
Ryvita — 4
Wasa Extra Crisp — 5
Wasa Fiber Plus — 5
Wasa Breakfast — 8

CROUTONS†
Croutons, cheese — 13
Croutons, onion or garlic — 16
Croutons, plain or seasoned — 20

FLOUR*
Flour, soy, full fat — 15
Flour, soy, defatted — 19
Flour, whole wheat — 44
Flour, white, unsifted — 48

MATZO AND MELBA†
Melba Toast, all flavors — 21
Matzo, egg — 23
Matzo, plain — 24

0   25   50   75   100
carbohydrates (grams)

* Counts are based on 1/2- cup servings.

** Counts are based on single item.

† Counts are based on single-ounce servings.

91

Bread, Crackers, and Flours:
PANCAKES, STUFFING & MORE*

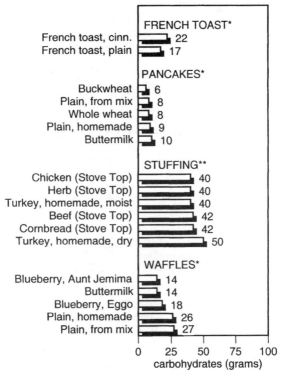

FRENCH TOAST*

French toast, cinn. — 22
French toast, plain — 17

PANCAKES*

Buckwheat — 6
Plain, from mix — 8
Whole wheat — 8
Plain, homemade — 9
Buttermilk — 10

STUFFING**

Chicken (Stove Top) — 40
Herb (Stove Top) — 40
Turkey, homemade, moist — 40
Beef (Stove Top) — 42
Cornbread (Stove Top) — 42
Turkey, homemade, dry — 50

WAFFLES*

Blueberry, Aunt Jemima — 14
Buttermilk — 14
Blueberry, Eggo — 18
Plain, homemade — 26
Plain, from mix — 27

0   25   50   75   100
carbohydrates (grams)

* Counts are based on a single slice, one pancake, or
  one waffle.
** Counts are based on 1/2-cup servings, prepared.

CEREALS*, Part 1

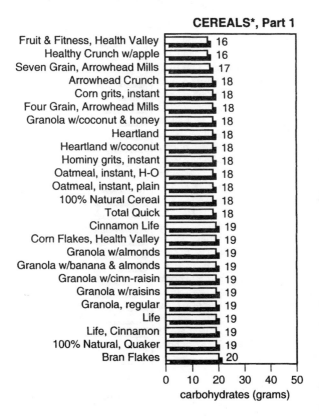

Cereal	carbohydrates (grams)
Fruit & Fitness, Health Valley	16
Healthy Crunch w/apple	16
Seven Grain, Arrowhead Mills	17
Arrowhead Crunch	18
Corn grits, instant	18
Four Grain, Arrowhead Mills	18
Granola w/coconut & honey	18
Heartland	18
Heartland w/coconut	18
Hominy grits, instant	18
Oatmeal, instant, H-O	18
Oatmeal, instant, plain	18
100% Natural Cereal	18
Total Quick	18
Cinnamon Life	19
Corn Flakes, Health Valley	19
Granola w/almonds	19
Granola w/banana & almonds	19
Granola w/cinn-raisin	19
Granola w/raisins	19
Granola, regular	19
Life	19
Life, Cinnamon	19
100% Natural, Quaker	19
Bran Flakes	20

carbohydrates (grams)

* Counts are based on average-size servings (as indicated
on package) and without added milk.

CEREALS*, Part 2

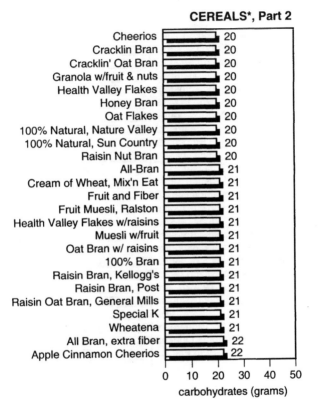

Cereal	carbohydrates (grams)
Cheerios	20
Cracklin Bran	20
Cracklin' Oat Bran	20
Granola w/fruit & nuts	20
Health Valley Flakes	20
Honey Bran	20
Oat Flakes	20
100% Natural, Nature Valley	20
100% Natural, Sun Country	20
Raisin Nut Bran	20
All-Bran	21
Cream of Wheat, Mix'n Eat	21
Fruit and Fiber	21
Fruit Muesli, Ralston	21
Health Valley Flakes w/raisins	21
Muesli w/fruit	21
Oat Bran w/ raisins	21
100% Bran	21
Raisin Bran, Kellogg's	21
Raisin Bran, Post	21
Raisin Oat Bran, General Mills	21
Special K	21
Wheatena	21
All Bran, extra fiber	22
Apple Cinnamon Cheerios	22

carbohydrates (grams)

* Counts are based on average-size servings (as indicated
  on package) and without added milk.

CEREALS*, Part 3

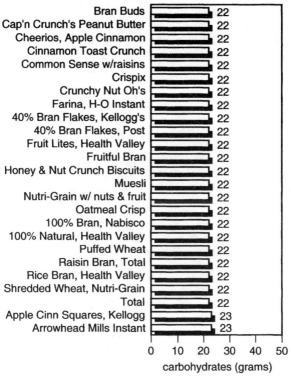

Cereal	carbohydrates (grams)
Bran Buds	22
Cap'n Crunch's Peanut Butter	22
Cheerios, Apple Cinnamon	22
Cinnamon Toast Crunch	22
Common Sense w/raisins	22
Crispix	22
Crunchy Nut Oh's	22
Farina, H-O Instant	22
40% Bran Flakes, Kellogg's	22
40% Bran Flakes, Post	22
Fruit Lites, Health Valley	22
Fruitful Bran	22
Honey & Nut Crunch Biscuits	22
Muesli	22
Nutri-Grain w/ nuts & fruit	22
Oatmeal Crisp	22
100% Bran, Nabisco	22
100% Natural, Health Valley	22
Puffed Wheat	22
Raisin Bran, Total	22
Rice Bran, Health Valley	22
Shredded Wheat, Nutri-Grain	22
Total	22
Apple Cinn Squares, Kellogg	23
Arrowhead Mills Instant	23

carbohydrates (grams)

* Counts are based on average-size servings (as indicated
on package) and without added milk.

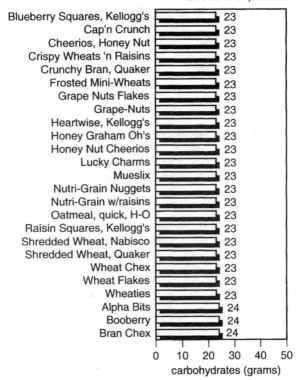

Hi-Low Comparison Chart
(for Alphabetical Charts, see pages 1 - 82)

CEREALS*, Part 4

Cereal	carbohydrates (grams)
Blueberry Squares, Kellogg's	23
Cap'n Crunch	23
Cheerios, Honey Nut	23
Crispy Wheats 'n Raisins	23
Crunchy Bran, Quaker	23
Frosted Mini-Wheats	23
Grape Nuts Flakes	23
Grape-Nuts	23
Heartwise, Kellogg's	23
Honey Graham Oh's	23
Honey Nut Cheerios	23
Lucky Charms	23
Mueslix	23
Nutri-Grain Nuggets	23
Nutri-Grain w/raisins	23
Oatmeal, quick, H-O	23
Raisin Squares, Kellogg's	23
Shredded Wheat, Nabisco	23
Shredded Wheat, Quaker	23
Wheat Chex	23
Wheat Flakes	23
Wheaties	23
Alpha Bits	24
Booberry	24
Bran Chex	24

carbohydrates (grams)

* Counts are based on average-size servings (as indicated
on package) and without added milk.

96

Hi-Low Comparison Chart
(for Alphabetical Charts, see pages 1 - 82)

CEREALS*, Part 5

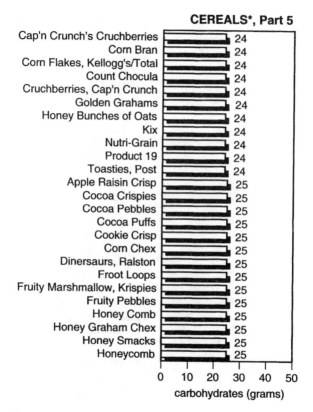

Cereal	carbohydrates (grams)
Cap'n Crunch's Cruchberries	24
Corn Bran	24
Corn Flakes, Kellogg's/Total	24
Count Chocula	24
Cruchberries, Cap'n Crunch	24
Golden Grahams	24
Honey Bunches of Oats	24
Kix	24
Nutri-Grain	24
Product 19	24
Toasties, Post	24
Apple Raisin Crisp	25
Cocoa Crispies	25
Cocoa Pebbles	25
Cocoa Puffs	25
Cookie Crisp	25
Corn Chex	25
Dinersaurs, Ralston	25
Froot Loops	25
Fruity Marshmallow, Krispies	25
Fruity Pebbles	25
Honey Comb	25
Honey Graham Chex	25
Honey Smacks	25
Honeycomb	25

carbohydrates (grams)

* Counts are based on average-size servings (as indicated
on package) and without added milk.

CEREALS*, Part 6

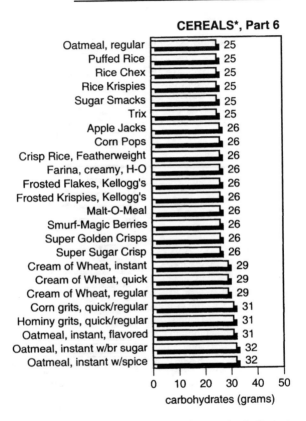

Cereal	carbohydrates (grams)
Oatmeal, regular	25
Puffed Rice	25
Rice Chex	25
Rice Krispies	25
Sugar Smacks	25
Trix	25
Apple Jacks	26
Corn Pops	26
Crisp Rice, Featherweight	26
Farina, creamy, H-O	26
Frosted Flakes, Kellogg's	26
Frosted Krispies, Kellogg's	26
Malt-O-Meal	26
Smurf-Magic Berries	26
Super Golden Crisps	26
Super Sugar Crisp	26
Cream of Wheat, instant	29
Cream of Wheat, quick	29
Cream of Wheat, regular	29
Corn grits, quick/regular	31
Hominy grits, quick/regular	31
Oatmeal, instant, flavored	31
Oatmeal, instant w/br sugar	32
Oatmeal, instant w/spice	32

carbohydrates (grams)

* Counts are based on average-size servings (as indicated
on package) and without added milk.

Hi-Low Comparison Chart
(for Alphabetical Charts, see pages 1 - 82)

COMBINED AND FROZEN FOODS*,
Part 1

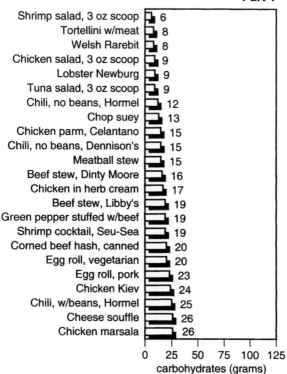

Food	carbohydrates (grams)
Shrimp salad, 3 oz scoop	6
Tortellini w/meat	8
Welsh Rarebit	8
Chicken salad, 3 oz scoop	9
Lobster Newburg	9
Tuna salad, 3 oz scoop	9
Chili, no beans, Hormel	12
Chop suey	13
Chicken parm, Celantano	15
Chili, no beans, Dennison's	15
Meatball stew	15
Beef stew, Dinty Moore	16
Chicken in herb cream	17
Beef stew, Libby's	19
Green pepper stuffed w/beef	19
Shrimp cocktail, Seu-Sea	19
Corned beef hash, canned	20
Egg roll, vegetarian	20
Egg roll, pork	23
Chicken Kiev	24
Chili, w/beans, Hormel	25
Cheese souffle	26
Chicken marsala	26

carbohydrates (grams)
0   25   50   75   100   125

* Counts are based on average-size servings as indicated
on package. Adjust count to reflect amount consumed.

COMBINED AND FROZEN FOOD

Par

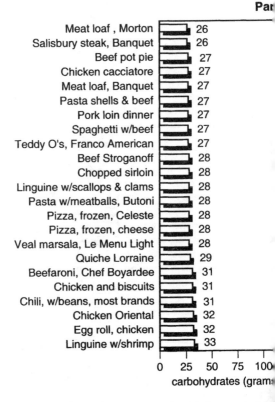

Food	carbohydrates (grams)
Meat loaf , Morton	26
Salisbury steak, Banquet	26
Beef pot pie	27
Chicken cacciatore	27
Meat loaf, Banquet	27
Pasta shells & beef	27
Pork loin dinner	27
Spaghetti w/beef	27
Teddy O's, Franco American	27
Beef Stroganoff	28
Chopped sirloin	28
Linguine w/scallops & clams	28
Pasta w/meatballs, Butoni	28
Pizza, frozen, Celeste	28
Pizza, frozen, cheese	28
Veal marsala, Le Menu Light	28
Quiche Lorraine	29
Beefaroni, Chef Boyardee	31
Chicken and biscuits	31
Chili, w/beans, most brands	31
Chicken Oriental	32
Egg roll, chicken	32
Linguine w/shrimp	33

0   25   50   75   100

carbohydrates (gram

* Counts are based on average-size servings as indica
on package. Adjust count to reflect amount consume

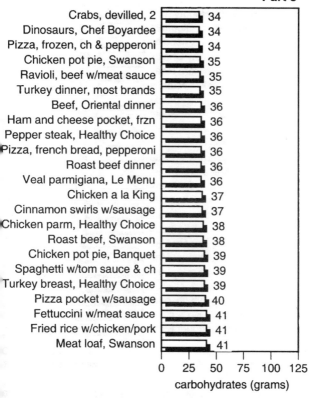

Hi-Low Comparison Chart
(for Alphabetical Charts, see pages 1 - 82)

**COMBINED AND FROZEN FOODS*,
Part 3**

Food	carbohydrates (grams)
Crabs, devilled, 2	34
Dinosaurs, Chef Boyardee	34
Pizza, frozen, ch & pepperoni	34
Chicken pot pie, Swanson	35
Ravioli, beef w/meat sauce	35
Turkey dinner, most brands	35
Beef, Oriental dinner	36
Ham and cheese pocket, frzn	36
Pepper steak, Healthy Choice	36
Pizza, french bread, pepperoni	36
Roast beef dinner	36
Veal parmigiana, Le Menu	36
Chicken a la King	37
Cinnamon swirls w/sausage	37
Chicken parm, Healthy Choice	38
Roast beef, Swanson	38
Chicken pot pie, Banquet	39
Spaghetti w/tom sauce & ch	39
Turkey breast, Healthy Choice	39
Pizza pocket w/sausage	40
Fettuccini w/meat sauce	41
Fried rice w/chicken/pork	41
Meat loaf, Swanson	41

0   25   50   75   100   125
carbohydrates (grams)

* Counts are based on average-size servings as indicated
on package. Adjust count to reflect amount consumed.

COMBINED AND FROZEN FOODS*, Part 4

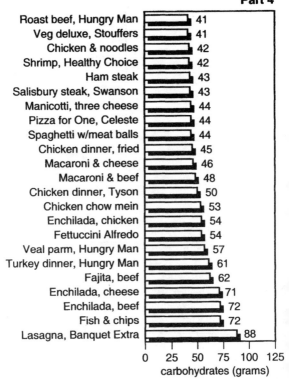

Food	carbohydrates (grams)
Roast beef, Hungry Man	41
Veg deluxe, Stouffers	41
Chicken & noodles	42
Shrimp, Healthy Choice	42
Ham steak	43
Salisbury steak, Swanson	43
Manicotti, three cheese	44
Pizza for One, Celeste	44
Spaghetti w/meat balls	44
Chicken dinner, fried	45
Macaroni & cheese	46
Macaroni & beef	48
Chicken dinner, Tyson	50
Chicken chow mein	53
Enchilada, chicken	54
Fettuccini Alfredo	54
Veal parm, Hungry Man	57
Turkey dinner, Hungry Man	61
Fajita, beef	62
Enchilada, cheese	71
Enchilada, beef	72
Fish & chips	72
Lasagna, Banquet Extra	88

0   25   50   75   100   125
carbohydrates (grams)

* Counts are based on average-size servings as indicated
on package. Adjust count to reflect amount consumed.

Dairy: CHEESE (HARD & SEMI-SOFT)*

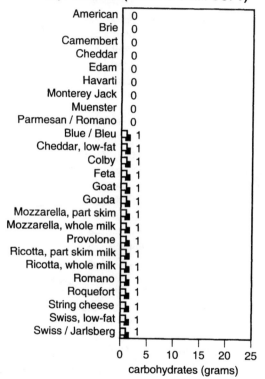

Cheese	carbohydrates (grams)
American	0
Brie	0
Camembert	0
Cheddar	0
Edam	0
Havarti	0
Monterey Jack	0
Muenster	0
Parmesan / Romano	0
Blue / Bleu	1
Cheddar, low-fat	1
Colby	1
Feta	1
Goat	1
Gouda	1
Mozzarella, part skim	1
Mozzarella, whole milk	1
Provolone	1
Ricotta, part skim milk	1
Ricotta, whole milk	1
Romano	1
Roquefort	1
String cheese	1
Swiss, low-fat	1
Swiss / Jarlsberg	1

carbohydrates (grams)

* Counts are based on one-ounce servings. Adjust count
to reflect amount consumed.

Dairy: CHEESES (SOFT), CREAMS & SUBSTITUTES*

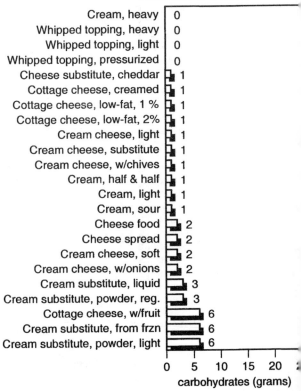

	carbohydrates (grams)
Cream, heavy	0
Whipped topping, heavy	0
Whipped topping, light	0
Whipped topping, pressurized	0
Cheese substitute, cheddar	1
Cottage cheese, creamed	1
Cottage cheese, low-fat, 1 %	1
Cottage cheese, low-fat, 2%	1
Cream cheese, light	1
Cream cheese, substitute	1
Cream cheese, w/chives	1
Cream, half & half	1
Cream, light	1
Cream, sour	1
Cheese food	2
Cheese spread	2
Cream cheese, soft	2
Cream cheese, w/onions	2
Cream substitute, liquid	3
Cream substitute, powder, reg.	3
Cottage cheese, w/fruit	6
Cream substitute, from frzn	6
Cream substitute, powder, light	6

* Counts are based on one-ounce servings of soft cheese
or one tablespoon of cream or whipped topping.

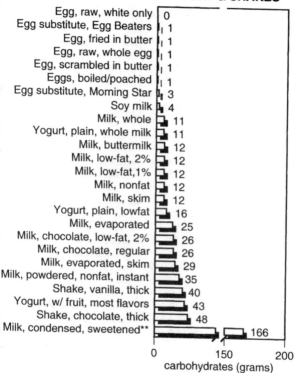

Hi-Low Comparison Chart
(for Alphabetical Charts, see pages 1 - 82)

Dairy: EGGS, MILK, YOGURT & SHAKES*

Item	carbohydrates (grams)
Egg, raw, white only	0
Egg substitute, Egg Beaters	1
Egg, fried in butter	1
Egg, raw, whole egg	1
Egg, scrambled in butter	1
Eggs, boiled/poached	1
Egg substitute, Morning Star	3
Soy milk	4
Milk, whole	11
Yogurt, plain, whole milk	11
Milk, buttermilk	12
Milk, low-fat, 2%	12
Milk, low-fat,1%	12
Milk, nonfat	12
Milk, skim	12
Yogurt, plain, lowfat	16
Milk, evaporated	25
Milk, chocolate, low-fat, 2%	26
Milk, chocolate, regular	26
Milk, evaporated, skim	29
Milk, powdered, nonfat, instant	35
Shake, vanilla, thick	40
Yogurt, w/ fruit, most flavors	43
Shake, chocolate, thick	48
Milk, condensed, sweetened**	166

carbohydrates (grams) — 0, 150, 200

* Counts based on one egg or equivalent egg substitute or 8 fluid ounces of milk, yogurt, or shake.
** High count for this item requires break in bar.

Dining Out: ASIAN*

Food	carbohydrates (grams)
Egg drop soup	6
Rice, sticky	7
Won ton soup, 2 won ton	11
Chicken, teriyaki	19
Egg roll, w/shrimp	21
Egg roll, vegetarian	23
Noodles, Japanese, udon	23
Noodles, Japanese, soba	24
Chop suey, w/beef & pork	26
Noodles, chow mein	26
Chow mein, w/beef or pork	32
Chow mein, w/chicken	32
Chow mein, w/shrimp	32
Chow mein, w/mushrooms	34
Chop suey	37
Chow mein, vegetarian	38
Green pepper steak	42
Beef, w/vegetables	48
Noodles, Japanese, somen	49
Rice, brown	50
Rice, white	50
Beef, w/broccoli	55
Beef, teriyaki	66
Chicken, sweet & sour	66
Pork, sweet & sour	66

carbohydrates (grams)

* Counts based on average-sized servings (for main dishes,
1 1/2 - 2 cups). Counts for main dishes include rice.

Dining Out: DELICATESSEN*

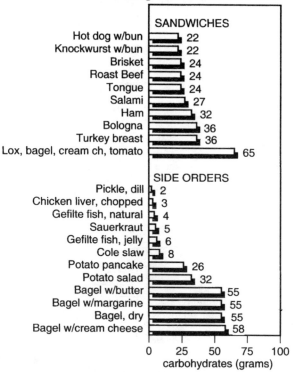

SANDWICHES

Hot dog w/bun	22
Knockwurst w/bun	22
Brisket	24
Roast Beef	24
Tongue	24
Salami	27
Ham	32
Bologna	36
Turkey breast	36
Lox, bagel, cream ch, tomato	65

SIDE ORDERS

Pickle, dill	2
Chicken liver, chopped	3
Gefilte fish, natural	4
Sauerkraut	5
Gefilte fish, jelly	6
Cole slaw	8
Potato pancake	26
Potato salad	32
Bagel w/butter	55
Bagel w/margarine	55
Bagel, dry	55
Bagel w/cream cheese	58

0   25   50   75   100
carbohydrates (grams)

* Unless otherwise indicated, counts based on average-
size servings or sandwiches. Sandwich counts assume
white or rye bread.

Dining Out: FRENCH AND
OTHER INTERNATIONAL DISHES*

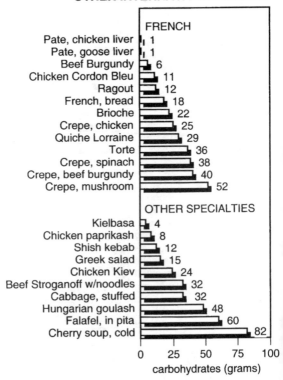

FRENCH

Pate, chicken liver	1
Pate, goose liver	1
Beef Burgundy	6
Chicken Cordon Bleu	11
Ragout	12
French, bread	18
Brioche	22
Crepe, chicken	25
Quiche Lorraine	29
Torte	36
Crepe, spinach	38
Crepe, beef burgundy	40
Crepe, mushroom	52

OTHER SPECIALTIES

Kielbasa	4
Chicken paprikash	8
Shish kebab	12
Greek salad	15
Chicken Kiev	24
Beef Stroganoff w/noodles	32
Cabbage, stuffed	32
Hungarian goulash	48
Falafel, in pita	60
Cherry soup, cold	82

0   25   50   75   100
carbohydrates (grams)

* Counts based on average-sized servings (for main dishes,
1 1/2 - 2 cups).

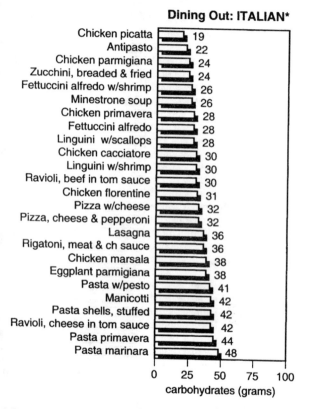

Hi-Low Comparison Chart
(for Alphabetical Charts, see pages 1 - 82)

Dining Out: ITALIAN*

Food	carbohydrates (grams)
Chicken picatta	19
Antipasto	22
Chicken parmigiana	24
Zucchini, breaded & fried	24
Fettuccini alfredo w/shrimp	26
Minestrone soup	26
Chicken primavera	28
Fettuccini alfredo	28
Linguini w/scallops	28
Chicken cacciatore	30
Linguini w/shrimp	30
Ravioli, beef in tom sauce	30
Chicken florentine	31
Pizza w/cheese	32
Pizza, cheese & pepperoni	32
Lasagna	36
Rigatoni, meat & ch sauce	36
Chicken marsala	38
Eggplant parmigiana	38
Pasta w/pesto	41
Manicotti	42
Pasta shells, stuffed	42
Ravioli, cheese in tom sauce	42
Pasta primavera	44
Pasta marinara	48

carbohydrates (grams)

* Counts are based on average-sized servings (1 1/2 - 2 cups); for pizza, on 1/6 medium or 1/8 large pizza).

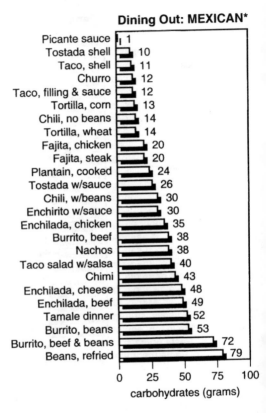

Dining Out: MEXICAN*

	carbohydrates (grams)
Picante sauce	1
Tostada shell	10
Taco, shell	11
Churro	12
Taco, filling & sauce	12
Tortilla, corn	13
Chili, no beans	14
Tortilla, wheat	14
Fajita, chicken	20
Fajita, steak	20
Plantain, cooked	24
Tostada w/sauce	26
Chili, w/beans	30
Enchirito w/sauce	30
Enchilada, chicken	35
Burrito, beef	38
Nachos	38
Taco salad w/salsa	40
Chimi	43
Enchilada, cheese	48
Enchilada, beef	49
Tamale dinner	52
Burrito, beans	53
Burrito, beef & beans	72
Beans, refried	79

* Counts based on average-sized servings (for main dishes,
1 1/2 - 2 cups).

Hi-Low Comparison Chart
(for Alphabetical Charts, see pages 1 - 82)

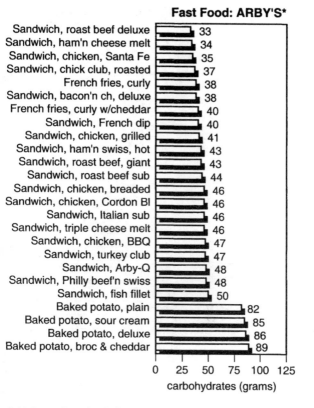

Fast Food: ARBY'S*

	carbohydrates (grams)
Sandwich, roast beef deluxe	33
Sandwich, ham'n cheese melt	34
Sandwich, chicken, Santa Fe	35
Sandwich, chick club, roasted	37
French fries, curly	38
Sandwich, bacon'n ch, deluxe	38
French fries, curly w/cheddar	40
Sandwich, French dip	40
Sandwich, chicken, grilled	41
Sandwich, ham'n swiss, hot	43
Sandwich, roast beef, giant	43
Sandwich, roast beef sub	44
Sandwich, chicken, breaded	46
Sandwich, chicken, Cordon Bl	46
Sandwich, Italian sub	46
Sandwich, triple cheese melt	46
Sandwich, chicken, BBQ	47
Sandwich, turkey club	47
Sandwich, Arby-Q	48
Sandwich, Philly beef'n swiss	48
Sandwich, fish fillet	50
Baked potato, plain	82
Baked potato, sour cream	85
Baked potato, deluxe	86
Baked potato, broc & cheddar	89

* Unless otherwise indicated, counts are based on average-
  size servings.

111

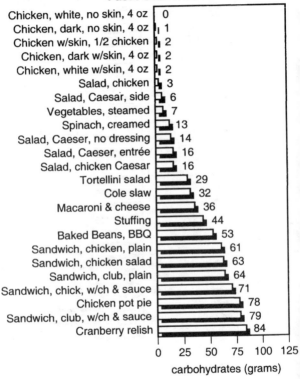

Hi-Low Comparison Chart
(for Alphabetical Charts, see pages 1 - 82)

Fast Food: BOSTON MARKET*

Item	carbohydrates (grams)
Chicken, white, no skin, 4 oz	0
Chicken, dark, no skin, 4 oz	1
Chicken w/skin, 1/2 chicken	2
Chicken, dark w/skin, 4 oz	2
Chicken, white w/skin, 4 oz	2
Salad, chicken	3
Salad, Caesar, side	6
Vegetables, steamed	7
Spinach, creamed	13
Salad, Caeser, no dressing	14
Salad, Caeser, entrée	16
Salad, chicken Caesar	16
Tortellini salad	29
Cole slaw	32
Macaroni & cheese	36
Stuffing	44
Baked Beans, BBQ	53
Sandwich, chicken, plain	61
Sandwich, chicken salad	63
Sandwich, club, plain	64
Sandwich, chick, w/ch & sauce	71
Chicken pot pie	78
Sandwich, club, w/ch & sauce	79
Cranberry relish	84

carbohydrates (grams)

* Unless otherwise indicated, counts are based on average-
size servings.

Fast Food: BURGER KING*

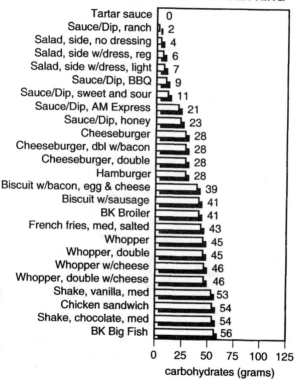

Item	carbohydrates (grams)
Tartar sauce	0
Sauce/Dip, ranch	2
Salad, side, no dressing	4
Salad, side w/dress, reg	6
Salad, side w/dress, light	7
Sauce/Dip, BBQ	9
Sauce/Dip, sweet and sour	11
Sauce/Dip, AM Express	21
Sauce/Dip, honey	23
Cheeseburger	28
Cheeseburger, dbl w/bacon	28
Cheeseburger, double	28
Hamburger	28
Biscuit w/bacon, egg & cheese	39
Biscuit w/sausage	41
BK Broiler	41
French fries, med, salted	43
Whopper	45
Whopper, double	45
Whopper w/cheese	46
Whopper, double w/cheese	46
Shake, vanilla, med	53
Chicken sandwich	54
Shake, chocolate, med	54
BK Big Fish	56

carbohydrates (grams)

* Unless otherwise indicated, counts are based on average-size servings.

Fast Food: HARDEE'S*

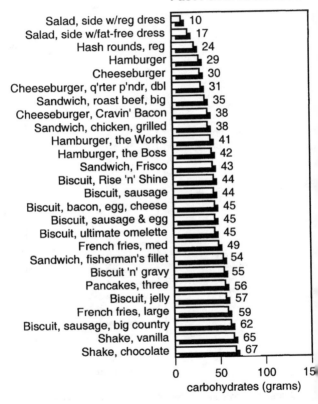

Item	carbohydrates (grams)
Salad, side w/reg dress	10
Salad, side w/fat-free dress	17
Hash rounds, reg	24
Hamburger	29
Cheeseburger	30
Cheeseburger, q'rter p'ndr, dbl	31
Sandwich, roast beef, big	35
Cheeseburger, Cravin' Bacon	38
Sandwich, chicken, grilled	38
Hamburger, the Works	41
Hamburger, the Boss	42
Sandwich, Frisco	43
Biscuit, Rise 'n' Shine	44
Biscuit, sausage	44
Biscuit, bacon, egg, cheese	45
Biscuit, sausage & egg	45
Biscuit, ultimate omelette	45
French fries, med	49
Sandwich, fisherman's fillet	54
Biscuit 'n' gravy	55
Pancakes, three	56
Biscuit, jelly	57
French fries, large	59
Biscuit, sausage, big country	62
Shake, vanilla	65
Shake, chocolate	67

carbohydrates (grams)

* Unless otherwise indicated, counts are based on average
size servings.

Fast Food: JACK IN THE BOX*

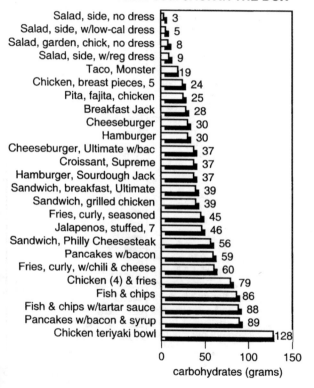

Item	carbohydrates (grams)
Salad, side, no dress	3
Salad, side, w/low-cal dress	5
Salad, garden, chick, no dress	8
Salad, side, w/reg dress	9
Taco, Monster	19
Chicken, breast pieces, 5	24
Pita, fajita, chicken	25
Breakfast Jack	28
Cheeseburger	30
Hamburger	30
Cheeseburger, Ultimate w/bac	37
Croissant, Supreme	37
Hamburger, Sourdough Jack	37
Sandwich, breakfast, Ultimate	39
Sandwich, grilled chicken	39
Fries, curly, seasoned	45
Jalapenos, stuffed, 7	46
Sandwich, Philly Cheesesteak	56
Pancakes w/bacon	59
Fries, curly, w/chili & cheese	60
Chicken (4) & fries	79
Fish & chips	86
Fish & chips w/tartar sauce	88
Pancakes w/bacon & syrup	89
Chicken teriyaki bowl	128

carbohydrates (grams)

* Unless otherwise indicated, counts are based on average-size servings.

Fast Food: KFC*

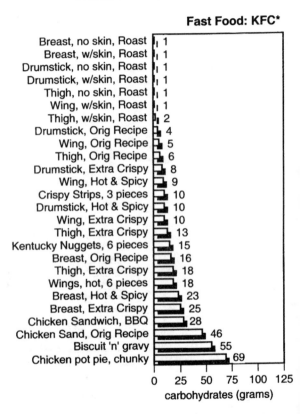

Breast, no skin, Roast	1
Breast, w/skin, Roast	1
Drumstick, no skin, Roast	1
Drumstick, w/skin, Roast	1
Thigh, no skin, Roast	1
Wing, w/skin, Roast	1
Thigh, w/skin, Roast	2
Drumstick, Orig Recipe	4
Wing, Orig Recipe	5
Thigh, Orig Recipe	6
Drumstick, Extra Crispy	8
Wing, Hot & Spicy	9
Crispy Strips, 3 pieces	10
Drumstick, Hot & Spicy	10
Wing, Extra Crispy	10
Thigh, Extra Crispy	13
Kentucky Nuggets, 6 pieces	15
Breast, Orig Recipe	16
Thigh, Extra Crispy	18
Wings, hot, 6 pieces	18
Breast, Hot & Spicy	23
Breast, Extra Crispy	25
Chicken Sandwich, BBQ	28
Chicken Sand, Orig Recipe	46
Biscuit 'n' gravy	55
Chicken pot pie, chunky	69

carbohydrates (grams)

* Unless otherwise indicated, counts are based on average-size servings.

Fast Food: MC DONALD'S*

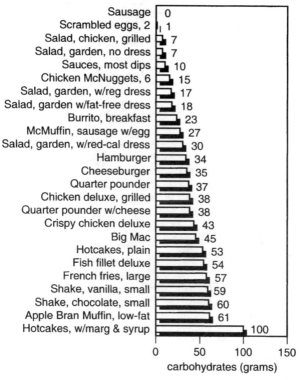

Food	carbohydrates (grams)
Sausage	0
Scrambled eggs, 2	1
Salad, chicken, grilled	7
Salad, garden, no dress	7
Sauces, most dips	10
Chicken McNuggets, 6	15
Salad, garden, w/reg dress	17
Salad, garden w/fat-free dress	18
Burrito, breakfast	23
McMuffin, sausage w/egg	27
Salad, garden, w/red-cal dress	30
Hamburger	34
Cheeseburger	35
Quarter pounder	37
Chicken deluxe, grilled	38
Quarter pounder w/cheese	38
Crispy chicken deluxe	43
Big Mac	45
Hotcakes, plain	53
Fish fillet deluxe	54
French fries, large	57
Shake, vanilla, small	59
Shake, chocolate, small	60
Apple Bran Muffin, low-fat	61
Hotcakes, w/marg & syrup	100

carbohydrates (grams)

* Unless otherwise indicated, counts are based on average-size servings.

117

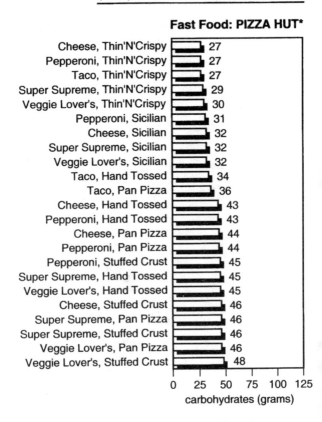

Hi-Low Comparison Chart
(for Alphabetical Charts, see pages 1 - 82)

Fast Food: PIZZA HUT*

	carbohydrates (grams)
Cheese, Thin'N'Crispy	27
Pepperoni, Thin'N'Crispy	27
Taco, Thin'N'Crispy	27
Super Supreme, Thin'N'Crispy	29
Veggie Lover's, Thin'N'Crispy	30
Pepperoni, Sicilian	31
Cheese, Sicilian	32
Super Supreme, Sicilian	32
Veggie Lover's, Sicilian	32
Taco, Hand Tossed	34
Taco, Pan Pizza	36
Cheese, Hand Tossed	43
Pepperoni, Hand Tossed	43
Cheese, Pan Pizza	44
Pepperoni, Pan Pizza	44
Pepperoni, Stuffed Crust	45
Super Supreme, Hand Tossed	45
Veggie Lover's, Hand Tossed	45
Cheese, Stuffed Crust	46
Super Supreme, Pan Pizza	46
Super Supreme, Stuffed Crust	46
Veggie Lover's, Pan Pizza	46
Veggie Lover's, Stuffed Crust	48

* Unless otherwise indicated, counts are based on average-size servings.

Fast Food: SUBWAY*

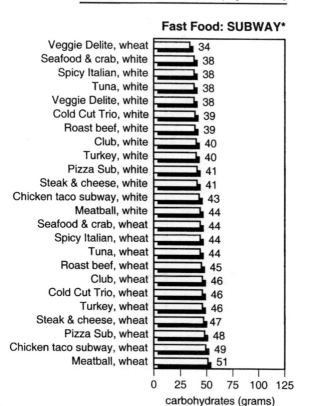

Item	carbohydrates (grams)
Veggie Delite, wheat	34
Seafood & crab, white	38
Spicy Italian, white	38
Tuna, white	38
Veggie Delite, white	38
Cold Cut Trio, white	39
Roast beef, white	39
Club, white	40
Turkey, white	40
Pizza Sub, white	41
Steak & cheese, white	41
Chicken taco subway, white	43
Meatball, white	44
Seafood & crab, wheat	44
Spicy Italian, wheat	44
Tuna, wheat	44
Roast beef, wheat	45
Club, wheat	46
Cold Cut Trio, wheat	46
Turkey, wheat	46
Steak & cheese, wheat	47
Pizza Sub, wheat	48
Chicken taco subway, wheat	49
Meatball, wheat	51

carbohydrates (grams)

* Unless otherwise indicated, counts are based on average-
size servings.

Hi-Low Comparison Chart
(for Alphabetical Charts, see pages 1 - 82)

Fast Food: TACO BELL*

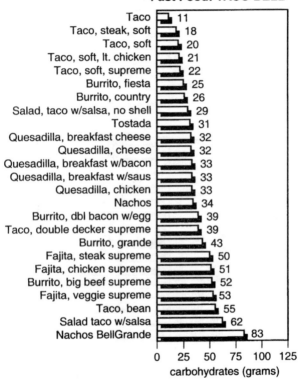

Item	carbohydrates (grams)
Taco	11
Taco, steak, soft	18
Taco, soft	20
Taco, soft, lt. chicken	21
Taco, soft, supreme	22
Burrito, fiesta	25
Burrito, country	26
Salad, taco w/salsa, no shell	29
Tostada	31
Quesadilla, breakfast cheese	32
Quesadilla, cheese	32
Quesadilla, breakfast w/bacon	33
Quesadilla, breakfast w/saus	33
Quesadilla, chicken	33
Nachos	34
Burrito, dbl bacon w/egg	39
Taco, double decker supreme	39
Burrito, grande	43
Fajita, steak supreme	50
Fajita, chicken supreme	51
Burrito, big beef supreme	52
Fajita, veggie supreme	53
Taco, bean	55
Salad taco w/salsa	62
Nachos BellGrande	83

* Unless otherwise indicated, counts are based on average-size servings.

Hi-Low Comparison Chart
(for Alphabetical Charts, see pages 1 - 82)

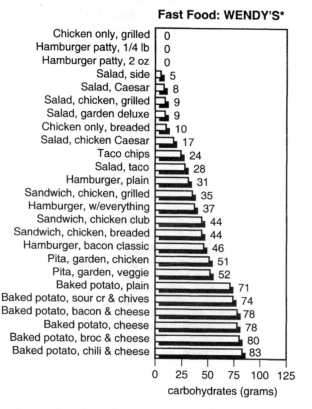

Fast Food: WENDY'S*

	carbohydrates (grams)
Chicken only, grilled	0
Hamburger patty, 1/4 lb	0
Hamburger patty, 2 oz	0
Salad, side	5
Salad, Caesar	8
Salad, chicken, grilled	9
Salad, garden deluxe	9
Chicken only, breaded	10
Salad, chicken Caesar	17
Taco chips	24
Salad, taco	28
Hamburger, plain	31
Sandwich, chicken, grilled	35
Hamburger, w/everything	37
Sandwich, chicken club	44
Sandwich, chicken, breaded	44
Hamburger, bacon classic	46
Pita, garden, chicken	51
Pita, garden, veggie	52
Baked potato, plain	71
Baked potato, sour cr & chives	74
Baked potato, bacon & cheese	78
Baked potato, cheese	78
Baked potato, broc & cheese	80
Baked potato, chili & cheese	83

carbohydrates (grams)

* Unless otherwise indicated, counts are based on average-size servings.

121

Fruits: FRESH & DRIED FRUITS AND JUICES *, Part 1

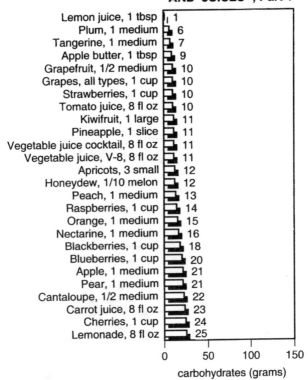

Food	carbohydrates (grams)
Lemon juice, 1 tbsp	1
Plum, 1 medium	6
Tangerine, 1 medium	7
Apple butter, 1 tbsp	9
Grapefruit, 1/2 medium	10
Grapes, all types, 1 cup	10
Strawberries, 1 cup	10
Tomato juice, 8 fl oz	10
Kiwifruit, 1 large	11
Pineapple, 1 slice	11
Vegetable juice cocktail, 8 fl oz	11
Vegetable juice, V-8, 8 fl oz	11
Apricots, 3 small	12
Honeydew, 1/10 melon	12
Peach, 1 medium	13
Raspberries, 1 cup	14
Orange, 1 medium	15
Nectarine, 1 medium	16
Blackberries, 1 cup	18
Blueberries, 1 cup	20
Apple, 1 medium	21
Pear, 1 medium	21
Cantaloupe, 1/2 medium	22
Carrot juice, 8 fl oz	23
Cherries, 1 cup	24
Lemonade, 8 fl oz	25

carbohydrates (grams)

* Unless otherwise indicated, counts are based on one whole, fresh fruit.

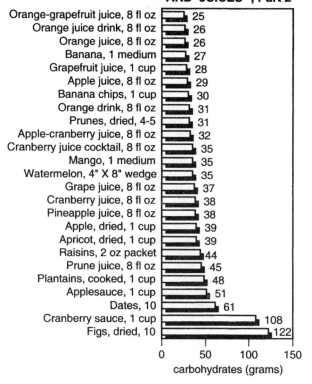

Hi-Low Comparison Chart
(for Alphabetical Charts, see pages 1 - 82)

Fruits: FRESH & DRIED FRUITS AND JUICES *, Part 2

Food	carbohydrates (grams)
Orange-grapefruit juice, 8 fl oz	25
Orange juice drink, 8 fl oz	26
Orange juice, 8 fl oz	26
Banana, 1 medium	27
Grapefruit juice, 1 cup	28
Apple juice, 8 fl oz	29
Banana chips, 1 cup	30
Orange drink, 8 fl oz	31
Prunes, dried, 4-5	31
Apple-cranberry juice, 8 fl oz	32
Cranberry juice cocktail, 8 fl oz	35
Mango, 1 medium	35
Watermelon, 4" X 8" wedge	35
Grape juice, 8 fl oz	37
Cranberry juice, 8 fl oz	38
Pineapple juice, 8 fl oz	38
Apple, dried, 1 cup	39
Apricot, dried, 1 cup	39
Raisins, 2 oz packet	44
Prune juice, 8 fl oz	45
Plantains, cooked, 1 cup	48
Applesauce, 1 cup	51
Dates, 10	61
Cranberry sauce, 1 cup	108
Figs, dried, 10	122

carbohydrates (grams)

* Unless otherwise indicated, counts are based on one whole, fresh fruit.

123

GRAVIES, SAUCES & DIPS*

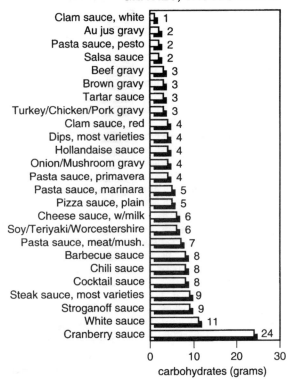

Food	carbohydrates (grams)
Clam sauce, white	1
Au jus gravy	2
Pasta sauce, pesto	2
Salsa sauce	2
Beef gravy	3
Brown gravy	3
Tartar sauce	3
Turkey/Chicken/Pork gravy	3
Clam sauce, red	4
Dips, most varieties	4
Hollandaise sauce	4
Onion/Mushroom gravy	4
Pasta sauce, primavera	4
Pasta sauce, marinara	5
Pizza sauce, plain	5
Cheese sauce, w/milk	6
Soy/Teriyaki/Worcestershire	6
Pasta sauce, meat/mush.	7
Barbecue sauce	8
Chili sauce	8
Cocktail sauce	8
Steak sauce, most varieties	9
Stroganoff sauce	9
White sauce	11
Cranberry sauce	24

carbohydrates (grams)

* Counts are based on one-quarter cup servings.

MEATS*, Part 1

	carbohydrates (grams)
BEEF	
Bottom round, lean	0
Bottom round, regular	0
Brisket, lean	0
Brisket, regular	0
Chuck, blade, lean	0
Chuck, blade, regular	0
Ground beef, lean	0
Ground beef, regular	0
Rib roast, lean	0
Rib roast, regular	0
Short ribs, lean	0
Short ribs, regular	0
Steak, sirloin, lean	0
Steak, sirloin, regular	0
Corned beef	1
LAMB	
Chops, arm, lean	0
Chops, arm, regular	0
Chops, loin, lean	0
Chops, loin, regular	0
Leg, lean	0
Leg, lean, regular	0
Rack rib, lean	0
Rack rib, regular	0

0   5   10   15   20   25

carbohydrates (grams)

* Counts are based on 3-ounce servings.

MEATS*, Part 2

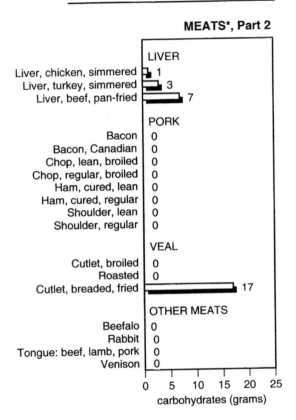

LIVER

Liver, chicken, simmered — 1
Liver, turkey, simmered — 3
Liver, beef, pan-fried — 7

PORK

Bacon — 0
Bacon, Canadian — 0
Chop, lean, broiled — 0
Chop, regular, broiled — 0
Ham, cured, lean — 0
Ham, cured, regular — 0
Shoulder, lean — 0
Shoulder, regular — 0

VEAL

Cutlet, broiled — 0
Roasted — 0
Cutlet, breaded, fried — 17

OTHER MEATS

Beefalo — 0
Rabbit — 0
Tongue: beef, lamb, pork — 0
Venison — 0

0   5   10   15   20   25
carbohydrates (grams)

* Counts are based on 3-ounce servings.

MEATS, PROCESSED*

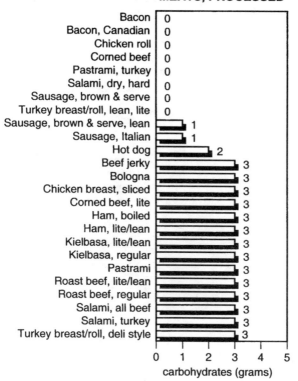

Item	carbohydrates (grams)
Bacon	0
Bacon, Canadian	0
Chicken roll	0
Corned beef	0
Pastrami, turkey	0
Salami, dry, hard	0
Sausage, brown & serve	0
Turkey breast/roll, lean, lite	0
Sausage, brown & serve, lean	1
Sausage, Italian	1
Hot dog	2
Beef jerky	3
Bologna	3
Chicken breast, sliced	3
Corned beef, lite	3
Ham, boiled	3
Ham, lite/lean	3
Kielbasa, lite/lean	3
Kielbasa, regular	3
Pastrami	3
Roast beef, lite/lean	3
Roast beef, regular	3
Salami, all beef	3
Salami, turkey	3
Turkey breast/roll, deli style	3

carbohydrates (grams)

* Counts are based on 3-ounce servings.

127

Medications: COUGH DROPS & SYRUPS*

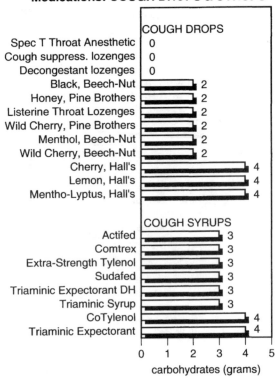

COUGH DROPS

	carbohydrates (grams)
Spec T Throat Anesthetic	0
Cough suppress. lozenges	0
Decongestant lozenges	0
Black, Beech-Nut	2
Honey, Pine Brothers	2
Listerine Throat Lozenges	2
Wild Cherry, Pine Brothers	2
Menthol, Beech-Nut	2
Wild Cherry, Beech-Nut	2
Cherry, Hall's	4
Lemon, Hall's	4
Mentho-Lyptus, Hall's	4

COUGH SYRUPS

	carbohydrates (grams)
Actifed	3
Comtrex	3
Extra-Strength Tylenol	3
Sudafed	3
Triaminic Expectorant DH	3
Triaminic Syrup	3
CoTylenol	4
Triaminic Expectorant	4

carbohydrates (grams)

* Counts are based on one cough drop or on recommended
doses for adults.

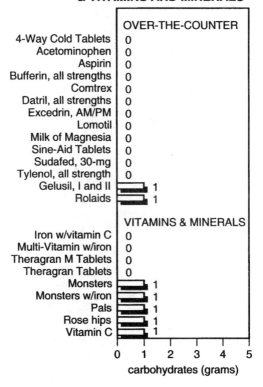

Hi-Low Comparison Chart
(for Alphabetical Charts, see pages 1 - 82)

Medications: OVER-THE-COUNTER REMEDIES & VITAMINS AND MINERALS*

OVER-THE-COUNTER

	carbohydrates (grams)
4-Way Cold Tablets	0
Acetominophen	0
Aspirin	0
Bufferin, all strengths	0
Comtrex	0
Datril, all strengths	0
Excedrin, AM/PM	0
Lomotil	0
Milk of Magnesia	0
Sine-Aid Tablets	0
Sudafed, 30-mg	0
Tylenol, all strength	0
Gelusil, I and II	1
Rolaids	1

VITAMINS & MINERALS

Iron w/vitamin C	0
Multi-Vitamin w/iron	0
Theragran M Tablets	0
Theragran Tablets	0
Monsters	1
Monsters w/iron	1
Pals	1
Rose hips	1
Vitamin C	1

carbohydrates (grams)

* Counts are based on recommended doses for adults.

129

MISCELLANEOUS FOODS*

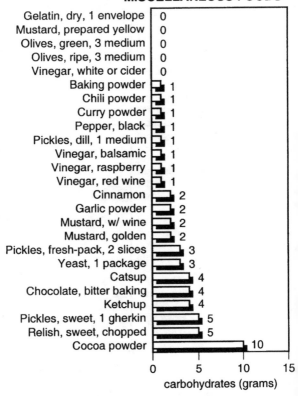

Food	carbohydrates (grams)
Gelatin, dry, 1 envelope	0
Mustard, prepared yellow	0
Olives, green, 3 medium	0
Olives, ripe, 3 medium	0
Vinegar, white or cider	0
Baking powder	1
Chili powder	1
Curry powder	1
Pepper, black	1
Pickles, dill, 1 medium	1
Vinegar, balsamic	1
Vinegar, raspberry	1
Vinegar, red wine	1
Cinnamon	2
Garlic powder	2
Mustard, w/ wine	2
Mustard, golden	2
Pickles, fresh-pack, 2 slices	3
Yeast, 1 package	3
Catsup	4
Chocolate, bitter baking	4
Ketchup	4
Pickles, sweet, 1 gherkin	5
Relish, sweet, chopped	5
Cocoa powder	10

carbohydrates (grams)

* Unless otherwise indicated, counts are based on a
one-tablespoon serving.

NUTS, BEANS AND SEEDS*: Part 1

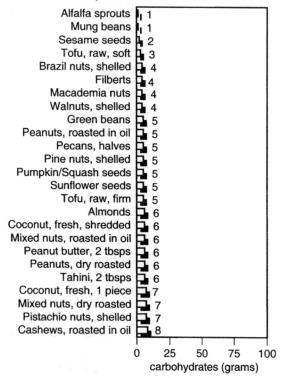

	carbohydrates (grams)
Alfalfa sprouts	1
Mung beans	1
Sesame seeds	2
Tofu, raw, soft	3
Brazil nuts, shelled	4
Filberts	4
Macadamia nuts	4
Walnuts, shelled	4
Green beans	5
Peanuts, roasted in oil	5
Pecans, halves	5
Pine nuts, shelled	5
Pumpkin/Squash seeds	5
Sunflower seeds	5
Tofu, raw, firm	5
Almonds	6
Coconut, fresh, shredded	6
Mixed nuts, roasted in oil	6
Peanut butter, 2 tbsps	6
Peanuts, dry roasted	6
Tahini, 2 tbsps	6
Coconut, fresh, 1 piece	7
Mixed nuts, dry roasted	7
Pistachio nuts, shelled	7
Cashews, roasted in oil	8

0   25   50   75   100
carbohydrates (grams)

* Unless otherwise indicated, counts are based on 1/2 cup
tofu or cooked beans or one-ounce servings of raw nuts or
seeds.

NUTS, BEANS AND SEEDS*: Part 2

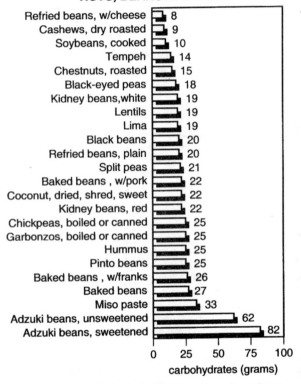

	carbohydrates (grams)
Refried beans, w/cheese	8
Cashews, dry roasted	9
Soybeans, cooked	10
Tempeh	14
Chestnuts, roasted	15
Black-eyed peas	18
Kidney beans, white	19
Lentils	19
Lima	19
Black beans	20
Refried beans, plain	20
Split peas	21
Baked beans , w/pork	22
Coconut, dried, shred, sweet	22
Kidney beans, red	22
Chickpeas, boiled or canned	25
Garbonzos, boiled or canned	25
Hummus	25
Pinto beans	25
Baked beans , w/franks	26
Baked beans	27
Miso paste	33
Adzuki beans, unsweetened	62
Adzuki beans, sweetened	82

* Unless otherwise indicated, counts are based on 1/2 cup
tofu or cooked beans or one-ounce servings of raw nuts or
seeds.

OILS AND FATS*

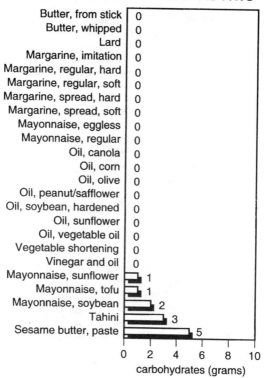

	carbohydrates (grams)
Butter, from stick	0
Butter, whipped	0
Lard	0
Margarine, imitation	0
Margarine, regular, hard	0
Margarine, regular, soft	0
Margarine, spread, hard	0
Margarine, spread, soft	0
Mayonnaise, eggless	0
Mayonnaise, regular	0
Oil, canola	0
Oil, corn	0
Oil, olive	0
Oil, peanut/safflower	0
Oil, soybean, hardened	0
Oil, sunflower	0
Oil, vegetable oil	0
Vegetable shortening	0
Vinegar and oil	0
Mayonnaise, sunflower	1
Mayonnaise, tofu	1
Mayonnaise, soybean	2
Tahini	3
Sesame butter, paste	5

* Counts are based on 1-tablespoon servings.

133

Hi-Low Comparison Chart
(for Alphabetical Charts, see pages 1 - 82)

PASTA, WHOLE GRAINS , RICE & NOODLES*, Part 1

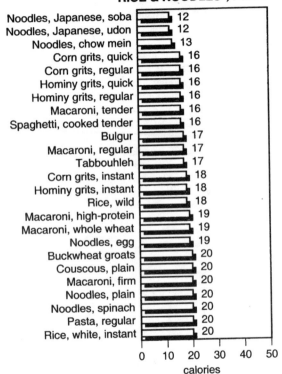

Food	calories
Noodles, Japanese, soba	12
Noodles, Japanese, udon	12
Noodles, chow mein	13
Corn grits, quick	16
Corn grits, regular	16
Hominy grits, quick	16
Hominy grits, regular	16
Macaroni, tender	16
Spaghetti, cooked tender	16
Bulgur	17
Macaroni, regular	17
Tabbouhleh	17
Corn grits, instant	18
Hominy grits, instant	18
Rice, wild	18
Macaroni, high-protein	19
Macaroni, whole wheat	19
Noodles, egg	19
Buckwheat groats	20
Couscous, plain	20
Macaroni, firm	20
Noodles, plain	20
Noodles, spinach	20
Pasta, regular	20
Rice, white, instant	20

* Counts are based on cooked, 1/2-cup servings.

PASTA, WHOLE GRAINS ,
RICE & NOODLES*, Part 2

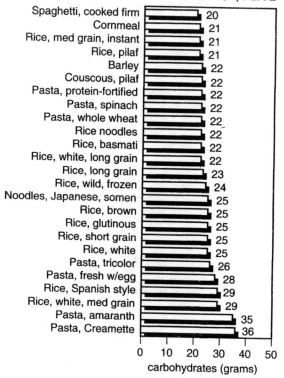

	carbohydrates (grams)
Spaghetti, cooked firm	20
Cornmeal	21
Rice, med grain, instant	21
Rice, pilaf	21
Barley	22
Couscous, pilaf	22
Pasta, protein-fortified	22
Pasta, spinach	22
Pasta, whole wheat	22
Rice noodles	22
Rice, basmati	22
Rice, white, long grain	22
Rice, long grain	23
Rice, wild, frozen	24
Noodles, Japanese, somen	25
Rice, brown	25
Rice, glutinous	25
Rice, short grain	25
Rice, white	25
Pasta, tricolor	26
Pasta, fresh w/egg	28
Rice, Spanish style	29
Rice, white, med grain	29
Pasta, amaranth	35
Pasta, Creamette	36

carbohydrates (grams)

* Counts are based on cooked, 1/2-cup servings.

Poultry: CHICKEN, TURKEY, AND OTHER FOWL*

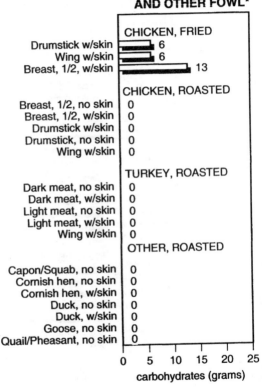

CHICKEN, FRIED

Drumstick w/skin	6
Wing w/skin	6
Breast, 1/2, w/skin	13

CHICKEN, ROASTED

Breast, 1/2, no skin	0
Breast, 1/2, w/skin	0
Drumstick w/skin	0
Drumstick, no skin	0
Wing w/skin	0

TURKEY, ROASTED

Dark meat, no skin	0
Dark meat, w/skin	0
Light meat, no skin	0
Light meat, w/skin	0
Wing w/skin	0

OTHER, ROASTED

Capon/Squab, no skin	0
Cornish hen, no skin	0
Cornish hen, w/skin	0
Duck, no skin	0
Duck, w/skin	0
Goose, no skin	0
Quail/Pheasant, no skin	0

0   5   10   15   20   25
carbohydrates (grams)

* Unless otherwise indicated, counts are based on 3-ounce servings.

SALAD BAR CHOICES*

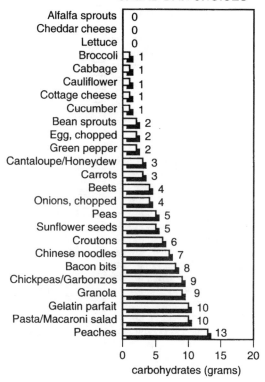

	carbohydrates (grams)
Alfalfa sprouts	0
Cheddar cheese	0
Lettuce	0
Broccoli	1
Cabbage	1
Cauliflower	1
Cottage cheese	1
Cucumber	1
Bean sprouts	2
Egg, chopped	2
Green pepper	2
Cantaloupe/Honeydew	3
Carrots	3
Beets	4
Onions, chopped	4
Peas	5
Sunflower seeds	5
Croutons	6
Chinese noodles	7
Bacon bits	8
Chickpeas/Garbonzos	9
Granola	9
Gelatin parfait	10
Pasta/Macaroni salad	10
Peaches	13

* Counts are based on one-quarter cup servings.

SALAD DRESSING*

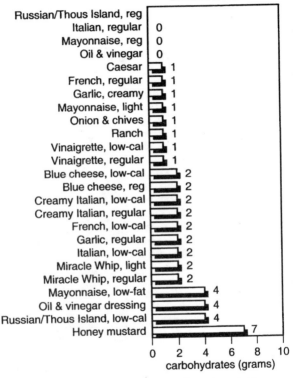

	carbohydrates (grams)
Russian/Thous Island, reg	
Italian, regular	0
Mayonnaise, reg	0
Oil & vinegar	0
Caesar	1
French, regular	1
Garlic, creamy	1
Mayonnaise, light	1
Onion & chives	1
Ranch	1
Vinaigrette, low-cal	1
Vinaigrette, regular	1
Blue cheese, low-cal	2
Blue cheese, reg	2
Creamy Italian, low-cal	2
Creamy Italian, regular	2
French, low-cal	2
Garlic, regular	2
Italian, low-cal	2
Miracle Whip, light	2
Miracle Whip, regular	2
Mayonnaise, low-fat	4
Oil & vinegar dressing	4
Russian/Thous Island, low-cal	4
Honey mustard	7

* For ease of comparison, counts are based on single
tablespoon servings. Adjust counts to reflect quantities
consumed.

Hi-Low Comparison Chart
(for Alphabetical Charts, see pages 1 - 82)

SEAFOOD*, Part 1

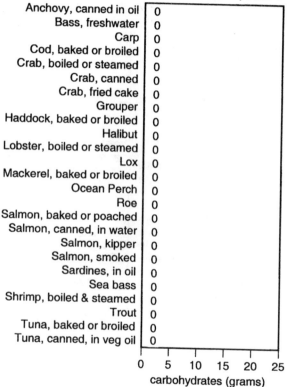

	carbohydrates (grams)
Anchovy, canned in oil	0
Bass, freshwater	0
Carp	0
Cod, baked or broiled	0
Crab, boiled or steamed	0
Crab, canned	0
Crab, fried cake	0
Grouper	0
Haddock, baked or broiled	0
Halibut	0
Lobster, boiled or steamed	0
Lox	0
Mackerel, baked or broiled	0
Ocean Perch	0
Roe	0
Salmon, baked or poached	0
Salmon, canned, in water	0
Salmon, kipper	0
Salmon, smoked	0
Sardines, in oil	0
Sea bass	0
Shrimp, boiled & steamed	0
Trout	0
Tuna, baked or broiled	0
Tuna, canned, in veg oil	0

0   5   10   15   20   25
carbohydrates (grams)

* Counts are based on 3-ounce servings. Canned seafood items are assumed to be drained.

SEAFOOD*, Part 2

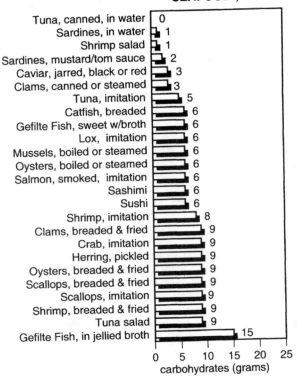

Food	carbohydrates (grams)
Tuna, canned, in water	0
Sardines, in water	1
Shrimp salad	1
Sardines, mustard/tom sauce	2
Caviar, jarred, black or red	3
Clams, canned or steamed	3
Tuna, imitation	5
Catfish, breaded	6
Gefilte Fish, sweet w/broth	6
Lox, imitation	6
Mussels, boiled or steamed	6
Oysters, boiled or steamed	6
Salmon, smoked, imitation	6
Sashimi	6
Sushi	6
Shrimp, imitation	8
Clams, breaded & fried	9
Crab, imitation	9
Herring, pickled	9
Oysters, breaded & fried	9
Scallops, breaded & fried	9
Scallops, imitation	9
Shrimp, breaded & fried	9
Tuna salad	9
Gefilte Fish, in jellied broth	15

carbohydrates (grams)

* Counts are based on 3-ounce servings. Canned seafood
items are assumed to be drained.

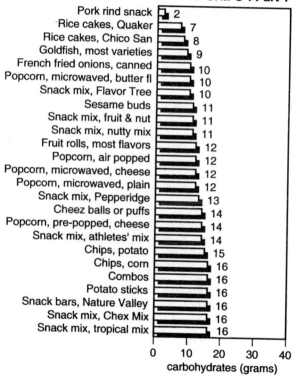

Hi-Low Comparison Chart
(for Alphabetical Charts, see pages 1 - 82)

SNACK FOODS AND CHIPS*: Part 1

Food	carbohydrates (grams)
Pork rind snack	2
Rice cakes, Quaker	7
Rice cakes, Chico San	8
Goldfish, most varieties	9
French fried onions, canned	10
Popcorn, microwaved, butter fl	10
Snack mix, Flavor Tree	10
Sesame buds	11
Snack mix, fruit & nut	11
Snack mix, nutty mix	11
Fruit rolls, most flavors	12
Popcorn, air popped	12
Popcorn, microwaved, cheese	12
Popcorn, microwaved, plain	12
Snack mix, Pepperidge	13
Cheez balls or puffs	14
Popcorn, pre-popped, cheese	14
Snack mix, athletes' mix	14
Chips, potato	15
Chips, corn	16
Combos	16
Potato sticks	16
Snack bars, Nature Valley	16
Snack mix, Chex Mix	16
Snack mix, tropical mix	16

0   10   20   30   40
carbohydrates (grams)

* For ease of comparison, counts are based on one-ounce servings. For popcorn, 1 ounce unpopped = 2 cups popped. Adjust count to reflect amount consumed.

141

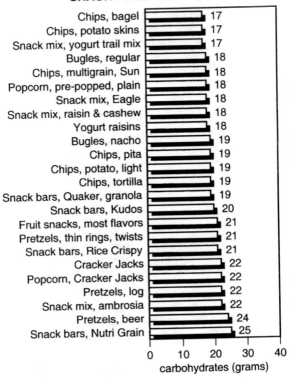

SNACK FOODS AND CHIPS*: Part 2

Food	carbohydrates (grams)
Chips, bagel	17
Chips, potato skins	17
Snack mix, yogurt trail mix	17
Bugles, regular	18
Chips, multigrain, Sun	18
Popcorn, pre-popped, plain	18
Snack mix, Eagle	18
Snack mix, raisin & cashew	18
Yogurt raisins	18
Bugles, nacho	19
Chips, pita	19
Chips, potato, light	19
Chips, tortilla	19
Snack bars, Quaker, granola	19
Snack bars, Kudos	20
Fruit snacks, most flavors	21
Pretzels, thin rings, twists	21
Snack bars, Rice Crispy	21
Cracker Jacks	22
Popcorn, Cracker Jacks	22
Pretzels, log	22
Snack mix, ambrosia	22
Pretzels, beer	24
Snack bars, Nutri Grain	25

carbohydrates (grams)

* For ease of comparison, counts are based on one-ounce
servings. For popcorn, 1 ounce unpopped = 2 cups popped.
Adjust count to reflect amount consumed.

SOUP*, Part 1

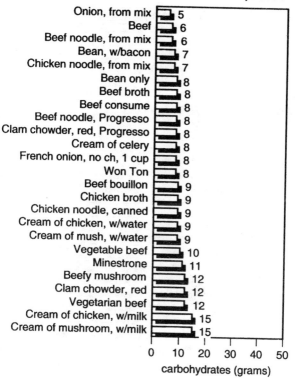

Food	carbohydrates (grams)
Onion, from mix	5
Beef	6
Beef noodle, from mix	6
Bean, w/bacon	7
Chicken noodle, from mix	7
Bean only	8
Beef broth	8
Beef consume	8
Beef noodle, Progresso	8
Clam chowder, red, Progresso	8
Cream of celery	8
French onion, no ch, 1 cup	8
Won Ton	8
Beef bouillon	9
Chicken broth	9
Chicken noodle, canned	9
Cream of chicken, w/water	9
Cream of mush, w/water	9
Vegetable beef	10
Minestrone	11
Beefy mushroom	12
Clam chowder, red	12
Vegetarian beef	12
Cream of chicken, w/milk	15
Cream of mushroom, w/milk	15

carbohydrates (grams)

* Unless otherwise indicated, counts are based on one-cup
servings.

143

Hi-Low Comparison Chart
(for Alphabetical Charts, see pages 1 - 82)

SOUP*, Part 2

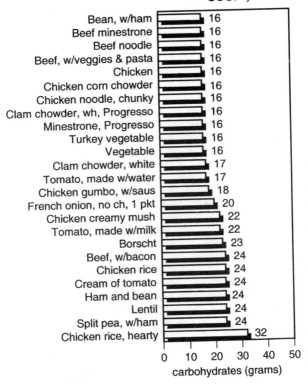

	carbohydrates (grams)
Bean, w/ham	16
Beef minestrone	16
Beef noodle	16
Beef, w/veggies & pasta	16
Chicken	16
Chicken corn chowder	16
Chicken noodle, chunky	16
Clam chowder, wh, Progresso	16
Minestrone, Progresso	16
Turkey vegetable	16
Vegetable	16
Clam chowder, white	17
Tomato, made w/water	17
Chicken gumbo, w/saus	18
French onion, no ch, 1 pkt	20
Chicken creamy mush	22
Tomato, made w/milk	22
Borscht	23
Beef, w/bacon	24
Chicken rice	24
Cream of tomato	24
Ham and bean	24
Lentil	24
Split pea, w/ham	24
Chicken rice, hearty	32

* Unless otherwise indicated, counts are based on one-cup
servings.

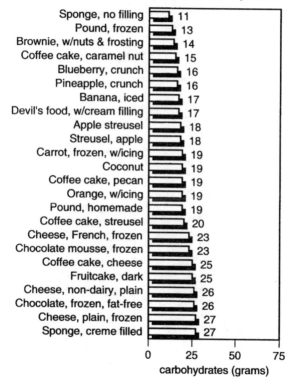

Hi-Low Comparison Chart
(for Alphabetical Charts, see pages 1 - 82)

Sweets: CAKES*, Part 1

Cake	carbohydrates (grams)
Sponge, no filling	11
Pound, frozen	13
Brownie, w/nuts & frosting	14
Coffee cake, caramel nut	15
Blueberry, crunch	16
Pineapple, crunch	16
Banana, iced	17
Devil's food, w/cream filling	17
Apple streusel	18
Streusel, apple	18
Carrot, frozen, w/icing	19
Coconut	19
Coffee cake, pecan	19
Orange, w/icing	19
Pound, homemade	19
Coffee cake, streusel	20
Cheese, French, frozen	23
Chocolate mousse, frozen	23
Coffee cake, cheese	25
Fruitcake, dark	25
Cheese, non-dairy, plain	26
Chocolate, frozen, fat-free	26
Cheese, plain, frozen	27
Sponge, creme filled	27

carbohydrates (grams)

* Counts are based on average-size pieces and slices,
where appropriate, as indicated on package.

Sweets: CAKES*, Part 2

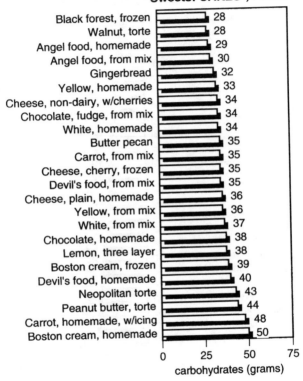

Food	carbohydrates (grams)
Black forest, frozen	28
Walnut, torte	28
Angel food, homemade	29
Angel food, from mix	30
Gingerbread	32
Yellow, homemade	33
Cheese, non-dairy, w/cherries	34
Chocolate, fudge, from mix	34
White, homemade	34
Butter pecan	35
Carrot, from mix	35
Cheese, cherry, frozen	35
Devil's food, from mix	35
Cheese, plain, homemade	36
Yellow, from mix	36
White, from mix	37
Chocolate, homemade	38
Lemon, three layer	38
Boston cream, frozen	39
Devil's food, homemade	40
Neopolitan torte	43
Peanut butter, torte	44
Carrot, homemade, w/icing	48
Boston cream, homemade	50

* Counts are based on average-size pieces and slices,
where appropriate, as indicated on package.

Sweets: SNACK CAKES*

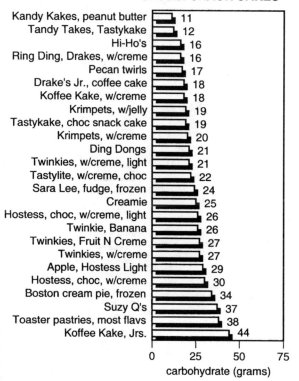

	carbohydrate (grams)
Kandy Kakes, peanut butter	11
Tandy Takes, Tastykake	12
Hi-Ho's	16
Ring Ding, Drakes, w/creme	16
Pecan twirls	17
Drake's Jr., coffee cake	18
Koffee Kake, w/creme	18
Krimpets, w/jelly	19
Tastykake, choc snack cake	19
Krimpets, w/creme	20
Ding Dongs	21
Twinkies, w/creme, light	21
Tastylite, w/creme, choc	22
Sara Lee, fudge, frozen	24
Creamie	25
Hostess, choc, w/creme, light	26
Twinkie, Banana	26
Twinkies, Fruit N Creme	27
Twinkies, w/creme	27
Apple, Hostess Light	29
Hostess, choc, w/creme	30
Boston cream pie, frozen	34
Suzy Q's	37
Toaster pastries, most flavs	38
Koffee Kake, Jrs.	44

* Counts based on serving size as indicated on package.

147

Sweets: CANDY*, Part 1

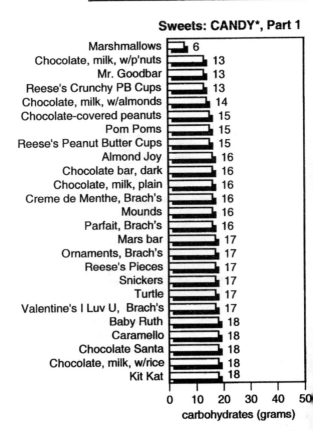

	carbohydrates (grams)
Marshmallows	6
Chocolate, milk, w/p'nuts	13
Mr. Goodbar	13
Reese's Crunchy PB Cups	13
Chocolate, milk, w/almonds	14
Chocolate-covered peanuts	15
Pom Poms	15
Reese's Peanut Butter Cups	15
Almond Joy	16
Chocolate bar, dark	16
Chocolate, milk, plain	16
Creme de Menthe, Brach's	16
Mounds	16
Parfait, Brach's	16
Mars bar	17
Ornaments, Brach's	17
Reese's Pieces	17
Snickers	17
Turtle	17
Valentine's I Luv U, Brach's	17
Baby Ruth	18
Caramello	18
Chocolate Santa	18
Chocolate, milk, w/rice	18
Kit Kat	18

* For ease of comparison, counts are based on one-ounce servings. Adjust counts to reflect quatities consumed.

Sweets: CANDY*, Part 2

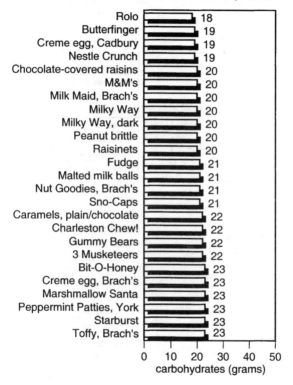

Candy	carbohydrates (grams)
Rolo	18
Butterfinger	19
Creme egg, Cadbury	19
Nestle Crunch	19
Chocolate-covered raisins	20
M&M's	20
Milk Maid, Brach's	20
Milky Way	20
Milky Way, dark	20
Peanut brittle	20
Raisinets	20
Fudge	21
Malted milk balls	21
Nut Goodies, Brach's	21
Sno-Caps	21
Caramels, plain/chocolate	22
Charleston Chew!	22
Gummy Bears	22
3 Musketeers	22
Bit-O-Honey	23
Creme egg, Brach's	23
Marshmallow Santa	23
Peppermint Patties, York	23
Starburst	23
Toffy, Brach's	23

carbohydrates (grams)

* For ease of comparison, counts are based on one-ounce
servings. Adjust counts to reflect quatities consumed.

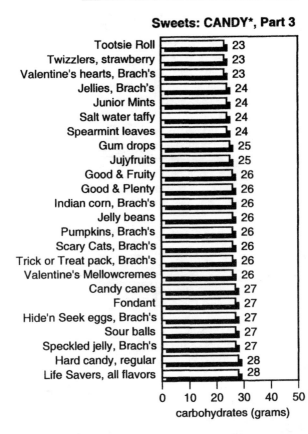

Hi-Low Comparison Chart
(for Alphabetical Charts, see pages 1 - 82)

Sweets: CANDY*, Part 3

	carbohydrates (grams)
Tootsie Roll	23
Twizzlers, strawberry	23
Valentine's hearts, Brach's	23
Jellies, Brach's	24
Junior Mints	24
Salt water taffy	24
Spearmint leaves	24
Gum drops	25
Jujyfruits	25
Good & Fruity	26
Good & Plenty	26
Indian corn, Brach's	26
Jelly beans	26
Pumpkins, Brach's	26
Scary Cats, Brach's	26
Trick or Treat pack, Brach's	26
Valentine's Mellowcremes	26
Candy canes	27
Fondant	27
Hide'n Seek eggs, Brach's	27
Sour balls	27
Speckled jelly, Brach's	27
Hard candy, regular	28
Life Savers, all flavors	28

* For ease of comparison, counts are based on one-ounce
servings. Adjust counts to reflect quatities consumed.

150

Sweets: COOKIES*, Part 1

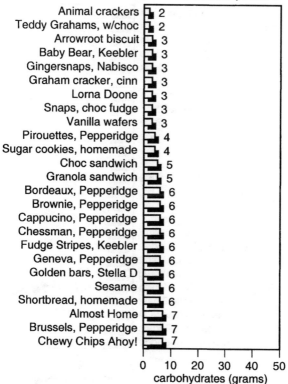

Cookie	carbohydrates (grams)
Animal crackers	2
Teddy Grahams, w/choc	2
Arrowroot biscuit	3
Baby Bear, Keebler	3
Gingersnaps, Nabisco	3
Graham cracker, cinn	3
Lorna Doone	3
Snaps, choc fudge	3
Vanilla wafers	3
Pirouettes, Pepperidge	4
Sugar cookies, homemade	4
Choc sandwich	5
Granola sandwich	5
Bordeaux, Pepperidge	6
Brownie, Pepperidge	6
Cappucino, Pepperidge	6
Chessman, Pepperidge	6
Fudge Stripes, Keebler	6
Geneva, Pepperidge	6
Golden bars, Stella D	6
Sesame	6
Shortbread, homemade	6
Almost Home	7
Brussels, Pepperidge	7
Chewy Chips Ahoy!	7

0 10 20 30 40 50
carbohydrates (grams)

* NOTE: For ease of comparison, counts are based on
single cookie servings. When more than one cookie is
consumed, counts should be adjusted accordingly.

151

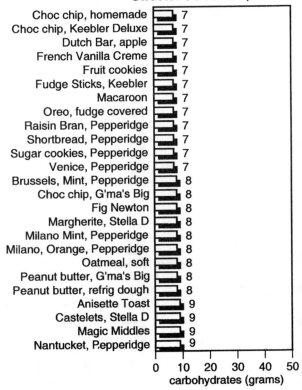

Hi-Low Comparison Chart
(for Alphabetical Charts, see pages 1 - 82)

Sweets: COOKIES*, Part 2

Choc chip, homemade	7
Choc chip, Keebler Deluxe	7
Dutch Bar, apple	7
French Vanilla Creme	7
Fruit cookies	7
Fudge Sticks, Keebler	7
Macaroon	7
Oreo, fudge covered	7
Raisin Bran, Pepperidge	7
Shortbread, Pepperidge	7
Sugar cookies, Pepperidge	7
Venice, Pepperidge	7
Brussels, Mint, Pepperidge	8
Choc chip, G'ma's Big	8
Fig Newton	8
Margherite, Stella D	8
Milano Mint, Pepperidge	8
Milano, Orange, Pepperidge	8
Oatmeal, soft	8
Peanut butter, G'ma's Big	8
Peanut butter, refrig dough	8
Anisette Toast	9
Castelets, Stella D	9
Magic Middles	9
Nantucket, Pepperidge	9

0   10   20   30   40   50
carbohydrates (grams)

* NOTE: For ease of comparison, counts are based on
single cookie servings. When more than one cookie is
consumed, counts should be adjusted accordingly.

Sweets: COOKIES*, Part 3

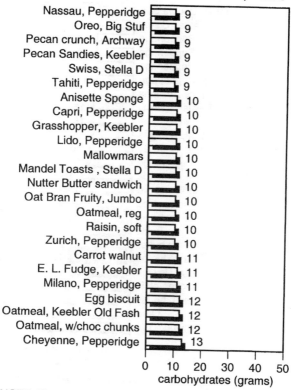

Cookie	carbohydrates (grams)
Nassau, Pepperidge	9
Oreo, Big Stuf	9
Pecan crunch, Archway	9
Pecan Sandies, Keebler	9
Swiss, Stella D	9
Tahiti, Pepperidge	9
Anisette Sponge	10
Capri, Pepperidge	10
Grasshopper, Keebler	10
Lido, Pepperidge	10
Mallowmars	10
Mandel Toasts , Stella D	10
Nutter Butter sandwich	10
Oat Bran Fruity, Jumbo	10
Oatmeal, reg	10
Raisin, soft	10
Zurich, Pepperidge	10
Carrot walnut	11
E. L. Fudge, Keebler	11
Milano, Pepperidge	11
Egg biscuit	12
Oatmeal, Keebler Old Fash	12
Oatmeal, w/choc chunks	12
Cheyenne, Pepperidge	13

carbohydrates (grams)

* NOTE: For ease of comparison, counts are based on
single cookie servings. When more than one cookie is
consumed, counts should be adjusted accordingly.

Sweets: COOKIES*, Part 4

Cookie	carbohydrates (grams)
Oreo, Double Stuf	13
Trolley Cakes	13
Beacon Hill, Pepperidge	14
Chantilly, Pepperidge	14
Chesapeake, Pepperidge	14
Sausalito, Pepperidge	14
Apple Newtons	15
Breakfast Treats, Stella D	15
Mystic Mint	15
Suddenly S'Mores	15
Gingersnaps, Archway	16
Santa Fe, Pepperidge	16
Choc chunk, homemade	19
Apple n'raisin	20
Chinese almond cookies	20
Pinwheels	20
Twirls	20
Peanut butter	22
Anisette Toast, Jumbo	23
Strawberry Newton	23
Graham cracker, plain	24
Graham cracker, honey	25
Oreo	33
Tastykake Bar	35

carbohydrates (grams)

* NOTE: For ease of comparison, counts are based on
single cookie servings. When more than one cookie is
consumed, counts should be adjusted accordingly.

Sweets: DONUTS*

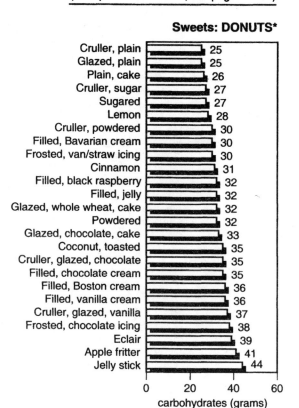

Donut	carbohydrates (grams)
Cruller, plain	25
Glazed, plain	25
Plain, cake	26
Cruller, sugar	27
Sugared	27
Lemon	28
Cruller, powdered	30
Filled, Bavarian cream	30
Frosted, van/straw icing	30
Cinnamon	31
Filled, black raspberry	32
Filled, jelly	32
Glazed, whole wheat, cake	32
Powdered	32
Glazed, chocolate, cake	33
Coconut, toasted	35
Cruller, glazed, chocolate	35
Filled, chocolate cream	35
Filled, Boston cream	36
Filled, vanilla cream	36
Cruller, glazed, vanilla	37
Frosted, chocolate icing	38
Eclair	39
Apple fritter	41
Jelly stick	44

carbohydrates (grams)

* Counts are based on average-size donuts.

155

Sweets: GUM & MINTS*

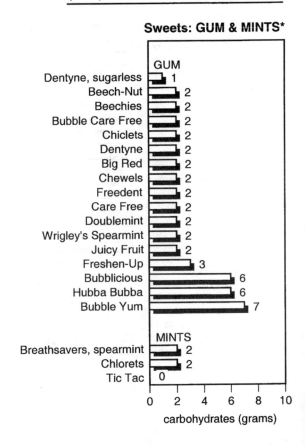

GUM

	carbohydrates (grams)
Dentyne, sugarless	1
Beech-Nut	2
Beechies	2
Bubble Care Free	2
Chiclets	2
Dentyne	2
Big Red	2
Chewels	2
Freedent	2
Care Free	2
Doublemint	2
Wrigley's Spearmint	2
Juicy Fruit	2
Freshen-Up	3
Bubblicious	6
Hubba Bubba	6
Bubble Yum	7

MINTS

Breathsavers, spearmint	2
Chlorets	2
Tic Tac	0

carbohydrates (grams)

* Counts are based on single sticks or mints.

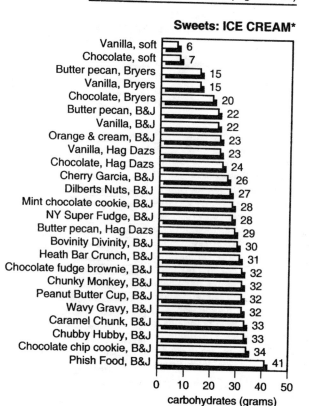

Hi-Low Comparison Chart
(for Alphabetical Charts, see pages 1 - 82)

Sweets: ICE CREAM*

	carbohydrates (grams)
Vanilla, soft	6
Chocolate, soft	7
Butter pecan, Bryers	15
Vanilla, Bryers	15
Chocolate, Bryers	20
Butter pecan, B&J	22
Vanilla, B&J	22
Orange & cream, B&J	23
Vanilla, Hag Dazs	23
Chocolate, Hag Dazs	24
Cherry Garcia, B&J	26
Dilberts Nuts, B&J	27
Mint chocolate cookie, B&J	28
NY Super Fudge, B&J	28
Butter pecan, Hag Dazs	29
Bovinity Divinity, B&J	30
Heath Bar Crunch, B&J	31
Chocolate fudge brownie, B&J	32
Chunky Monkey, B&J	32
Peanut Butter Cup, B&J	32
Wavy Gravy, B&J	32
Caramel Chunk, B&J	33
Chubby Hubby, B&J	33
Chocolate chip cookie, B&J	34
Phish Food, B&J	41

0 10 20 30 40 50
carbohydrates (grams)

* Counts are based on one-half cup servings. "B&J"
designates Ben & Jerry's brand.

157

Sweets: ICE CREAM CONES & BARS, ICE CREAM ALTERNATIVES AND PUDDINGS*

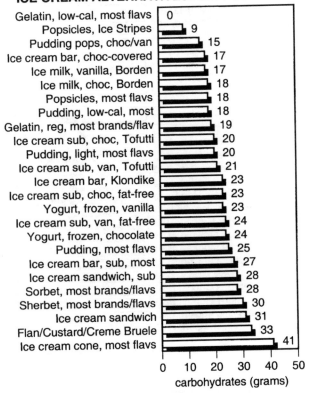

Item	carbohydrates (grams)
Gelatin, low-cal, most flavs	0
Popsicles, Ice Stripes	9
Pudding pops, choc/van	15
Ice cream bar, choc-covered	17
Ice milk, vanilla, Borden	17
Ice milk, choc, Borden	18
Popsicles, most flavs	18
Pudding, low-cal, most	18
Gelatin, reg, most brands/flav	19
Ice cream sub, choc, Tofutti	20
Pudding, light, most flavs	20
Ice cream sub, van, Tofutti	21
Ice cream bar, Klondike	23
Ice cream sub, choc, fat-free	23
Yogurt, frozen, vanilla	23
Ice cream sub, van, fat-free	24
Yogurt, frozen, chocolate	24
Pudding, most flavs	25
Ice cream bar, sub, most	27
Ice cream sandwich, sub	28
Sorbet, most brands/flavs	28
Sherbet, most brands/flavs	30
Ice cream sandwich	31
Flan/Custard/Creme Bruele	33
Ice cream cone, most flavs	41

carbohydrates (grams)

* Counts are based on average- or one-half cup servings.
"Sub" designates non-dairy, ice cream substitute.

158

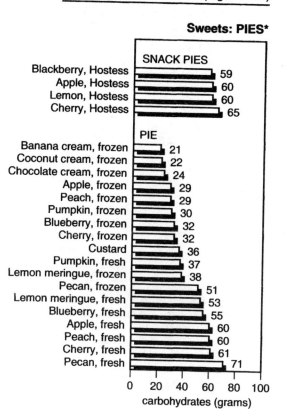

Sweets: PIES*

SNACK PIES

	carbohydrates (grams)
Blackberry, Hostess	59
Apple, Hostess	60
Lemon, Hostess	60
Cherry, Hostess	65

PIE

	carbohydrates (grams)
Banana cream, frozen	21
Coconut cream, frozen	22
Chocolate cream, frozen	24
Apple, frozen	29
Peach, frozen	29
Pumpkin, frozen	30
Blueberry, frozen	32
Cherry, frozen	32
Custard	36
Pumpkin, fresh	37
Lemon meringue, frozen	38
Pecan, frozen	51
Lemon meringue, fresh	53
Blueberry, fresh	55
Apple, fresh	60
Peach, fresh	60
Cherry, fresh	61
Pecan, fresh	71

carbohydrates (grams)

* Counts are based on average-size pieces and slices,
where appropriate, as indicated on package.

Sweets: SUGARS, SYRUPS, TOPPINGS AND JAMS*

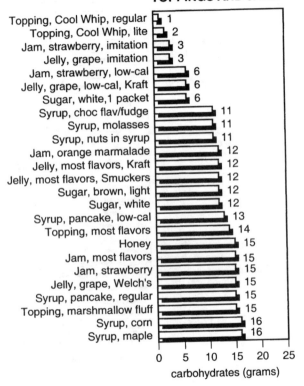

Item	carbohydrates (grams)
Topping, Cool Whip, regular	1
Topping, Cool Whip, lite	2
Jam, strawberry, imitation	3
Jelly, grape, imitation	3
Jam, strawberry, low-cal	6
Jelly, grape, low-cal, Kraft	6
Sugar, white, 1 packet	6
Syrup, choc flav/fudge	11
Syrup, molasses	11
Syrup, nuts in syrup	11
Jam, orange marmalade	12
Jelly, most flavors, Kraft	12
Jelly, most flavors, Smuckers	12
Sugar, brown, light	12
Sugar, white	12
Syrup, pancake, low-cal	13
Topping, most flavors	14
Honey	15
Jam, most flavors	15
Jam, strawberry	15
Jelly, grape, Welch's	15
Syrup, pancake, regular	15
Topping, marshmallow fluff	15
Syrup, corn	16
Syrup, maple	16

carbohydrates (grams)

* Counts are based on single-tablespoon servings. Jams and preserves can be assumed to have equal values.

VEGETABLES*, Part 1

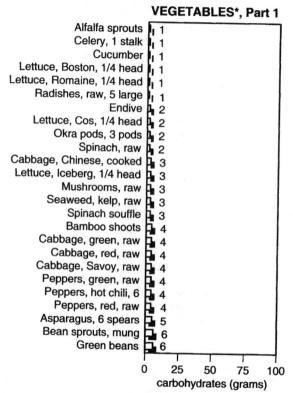

	carbohydrates (grams)
Alfalfa sprouts	1
Celery, 1 stalk	1
Cucumber	1
Lettuce, Boston, 1/4 head	1
Lettuce, Romaine, 1/4 head	1
Radishes, raw, 5 large	1
Endive	2
Lettuce, Cos, 1/4 head	2
Okra pods, 3 pods	2
Spinach, raw	2
Cabbage, Chinese, cooked	3
Lettuce, Iceberg, 1/4 head	3
Mushrooms, raw	3
Seaweed, kelp, raw	3
Spinach souffle	3
Bamboo shoots	4
Cabbage, green, raw	4
Cabbage, red, raw	4
Cabbage, Savoy, raw	4
Peppers, green, raw	4
Peppers, hot chili, 6	4
Peppers, red, raw	4
Asparagus, 6 spears	5
Bean sprouts, mung	6
Green beans	6

0 25 50 75 100
carbohydrates (grams)

* Unless otherwise indicated, counts are based on one-cup servings. For vegetable juices, see the Fruits & Juices section.

VEGETABLES*, Part 2

Food	carbohydrates (grams)
Cauliflower	6
Eggplant	6
Mung bean, sprouted	6
Turnip greens	6
Cabbage, green, cooked	7
Carrots, raw	7
Greens	7
Kale	7
Seaweed, Spirulina, dried	7
Broccoli, 1 spear	8
Mushrooms, boiled/canned	8
Spinach, cooked	8
Squash, summer, cooked	8
Tomato, raw, 1 large	8
Turnips, cooked	8
Sauerkraut	10
Tomatoes, canned	10
Beets	11
Kohlrabi, stems	11
Pea pods, Chinese, cooked	11
Artichokes, 1 large	12
Onions, raw	12
Brussels sprouts	13
Onions, cooked	13
Carrots, cooked	16

carbohydrates (grams): 0   25   50   75   100

* Unless otherwise indicated, counts are based on one-cup
servings. For vegetable juices, see the Fruits & Juices
section.

VEGETABLES*, Part 3

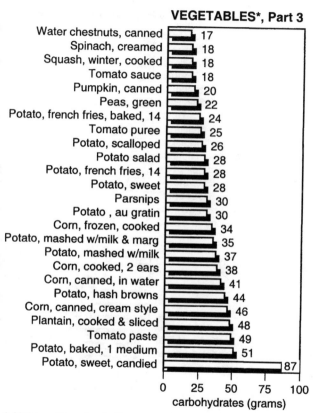

Food	carbohydrates (grams)
Water chestnuts, canned	17
Spinach, creamed	18
Squash, winter, cooked	18
Tomato sauce	18
Pumpkin, canned	20
Peas, green	22
Potato, french fries, baked, 14	24
Tomato puree	25
Potato, scalloped	26
Potato salad	28
Potato, french fries, 14	28
Potato, sweet	28
Parsnips	30
Potato , au gratin	30
Corn, frozen, cooked	34
Potato, mashed w/milk & marg	35
Potato, mashed w/milk	37
Corn, cooked, 2 ears	38
Corn, canned, in water	41
Potato, hash browns	44
Corn, canned, cream style	46
Plantain, cooked & sliced	48
Tomato paste	49
Potato, baked, 1 medium	51
Potato, sweet, candied	87

carbohydrates (grams)

* Unless otherwise indicated, counts are based on one-cup
servings. For vegetable juices, see the Fruits & Juices
section.

VEGETARIAN CHOICES*

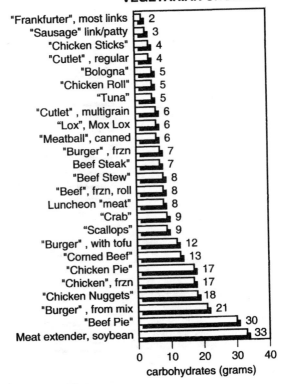

	carbohydrates (grams)
"Frankfurter", most links	2
"Sausage" link/patty	3
"Chicken Sticks"	4
"Cutlet", regular	4
"Bologna"	5
"Chicken Roll"	5
"Tuna"	5
"Cutlet", multigrain	6
"Lox", Mox Lox	6
"Meatball", canned	6
"Burger", frzn	7
Beef Steak"	7
"Beef Stew"	8
"Beef", frzn, roll	8
Luncheon "meat"	8
"Crab"	9
"Scallops"	9
"Burger", with tofu	12
"Corned Beef"	13
"Chicken Pie"	17
"Chicken", frzn	17
"Chicken Nuggets"	18
"Burger", from mix	21
"Beef Pie"	30
Meat extender, soybean	33

carbohydrates (grams)

* Made from tofu, textured vegetable protein or a combination of both. Counts are based on 3-ounce servings.